MW00861969

Succeeding in the Practicum

A Preparation Guide for Medical Assisting and Allied Health

THIRD EDITION

Succeeding in the Practicum

A Preparation Guide for Medical Assisting and Allied Health

Kim Bender, MS

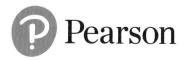 Pearson

Senior Vice President, Portfolio Management: Adam Jaworski
Director of Portfolio Management: Marlene McHugh Pratt
Portfolio Management Assistant: Emily Edling
Vice President, Content Production and Digital Studio: Paul DeLuca
Managing Producer, Health Science: Melissa Bashe
Content Producer: Faye Gemmellaro
Editorial Project Manager: Katherine Tiffany Ragay, SPi Global
Full-Service Project Manager: Subash Raju, SPi Global
Operations Specialist: Maura Zaldivar-Garcia
Creative Digital Lead: Mary Siener
Director, Digital Production: Amy Peltier

Digital Studio Producer, REVEL and eText 2.0: Ellen Viagnola
Digital Content Team Lead: Brian Prybella
Digital Content Project Lead: Lisa Rinaldi
Vice President, Product Marketing: Brad Parkins
Product Marketing Manager: Rachele Strober
Senior Field Marketing Manager: Brittany Hammond
Full Service Project Management and Composition: SPi Global
Inventory Manager: Vatche Demirdjian
Interior Design: Pearson CSC
Cover Design: Pearson CSC
Cover Art: Hero Images/Getty Images
Printer/Binder: LSC Communications, Inc.
Cover Printer: Phoenix Color Hagerstown

Credits and acknowledgments for material borrowed from other sources and reproduced, with permission, in this textbook appear on the appropriate page within the text.

Copyright © 2020 by Pearson Education, Inc. 221 River Street, Hoboken, NJ 07030. All rights reserved. Manufactured in the United States of America. This publication is protected by Copyright, and permission should be obtained from the publisher prior to any prohibited reproduction, storage in a retrieval system, or transmission in any form or by any means, electronic, mechanical, photocopying, recording, or likewise. To obtain permission(s) to use material from this work, please submit a written request to Pearson Education, Inc., Permissions Department, One Lake Street, Upper Saddle River, New Jersey 07458, or you may fax your request to 201-236-3290.

Note: Previous editions of this book were published under the title *Excelling in the Externship: A Preparation Guide for Medical Assisting and Allied Health*

Library of Congress Control Number: 2018044820

Names: Bender, Kim (Kimberly), author.
Title: Succeeding in the practicum : a preparation guide for medical assisting and allied health / Kim Bender.
Other titles: Excelling in the externship.
Description: 3rd edition. | Boston : Pearson, [2020] | Preceded by Excelling in the externship : a preparation guide for medical assisting and allied health / Kimberly Halverson-Bender. 2nd edition. 2014. | Includes bibliographical references and index.
Identifiers: LCCN 2018044820| ISBN 9780134874203 (alk. paper) | ISBN 013487420X (alk. paper)
Subjects: | MESH: Allied Health Personnel—education | Clinical Competence | Vocational Guidance | Preceptorship
Classification: LCC R847 | NLM W 18 | DDC 610.73/7069—dc23 LC record available at https://lccn.loc.gov/2018044820

1 19

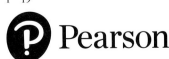

ISBN 10: 0-13-487420X
ISBN 13: 978-013-4874203

Contents

Chapter Five: Etiquette and Professional Manners   54

Chapter Six: Communication and Developing Professional Relationships   66

Chapter Seven: Fulfilling the "Student" Role During the Practicum   82

Chapter Eight: Benefits of Successful Practicum Completion   93

Chapter Nine: Performance Evaluation and Your Grade   102

Preface

The title of this edition has been changed from *Excelling in the Externship* to *Succeeding in the Practicum* to reflect the updated terminology used by the American Association of Medical Assistants to refer to the off-site training component of accredited Medical Assisting and other allied health programs. This title change puts us in line with the accrediting bodies and professional organizations.

The progression from completing the allied health program of study to becoming a professional within the industry is bridged by the practicum. This practicum encompasses the time and place in which the student has the opportunity to begin building professional relationships and to show off his or her technical skills and unique talents in serving and working with others. It is a time when avoidable pitfalls should not interfere with various professional opportunities. To make the most of the practicum, students must be well-prepared to take on new challenges, act responsibly, learn proactively, and develop themselves professionally, which are all major goals of *Succeeding in the Practicum*.

The overall purpose of *Succeeding in the Practicum* is to present to students the full picture of the practicum experience. Student readers will realize the value and purpose of the practicum, will be prepared by being familiar with the expectations for all aspects of the journey, and will discover the benefits and opportunities that await them when they begin their careers with completion of a successful practicum. They also will be given tips on the various pitfalls and mistakes to avoid in order to excel in the practicum. Coverage of the practicum from preterm to postterm is provided to guide students' focus and to help them maintain professionalism, responsibility, a positive attitude, and proactive learning throughout the process. The goal of this text is to prepare allied health students for a successful practical experience. In turn, this helps student-graduates to launch their careers with confidence, motivation, and meaningful experience. This also helps educational institutions send well-prepared students who intend to succeed to their partnering or affiliated offices, hospitals, pharmacies, and other facilities.

The content covered in this text is based on a significant amount of experience I have had with students and their practicums, which makes this worthwhile reading for any budding allied health professional approaching the practicum phase. Many colleges and educational institutions may offer, or do not provide, very limited preparation for students in the specific, yet important, aspects of switching on the professionalism required in allied health fields, which actually must begin before or during the practicum. This guide is intended to fill this gap in practicum preparation when significant face-to-face time between instructors and students for this purpose is unachievable within the established curriculum. It can be used concurrently with other related course material or as an independent study for students prior to beginning a practicum.

Succeeding in the Practicum is organized logically, beginning with introducing the purpose and value of the practicum. The text then maps out what the practicum site staff and the college or school expects of students. A chapter about practicum interviews focuses on preparing students who are required to attend an interview prior to beginning the practicum. Appropriate attitudes, etiquette, and the development of working professional relationships are discussed.

Next, how students are to fulfill the student role through following instructions and engaging in proactive learning is explored. Meant to serve as motivation for students, the next section discusses the priceless benefits of completing a practicum, some of which are tied to the specific training site. Material covering practicum evaluations and grades touches on the conclusion of the practicum phase. Real-life case studies follow. The final chapter explores the beginning of the job search for allied health careers.

Features of This Text

- **Tips from Professionals.** Brief sections throughout this guide provide up-front, practical advice. This is one of the most valuable features of this text. These insights based on the general experiences of industry professionals support the many topics in this text while providing information and recommendations.

- **Self-Prep Questions.** These questions are provided to guide and prepare students for each aspect of their practicum experience. They prompt students to think about what they will do when put into certain situations, as well as how to evaluate and improve their performance. An example from Chapter 3 preps students by requiring them to think of questions to ask in an interview, while examples in Chapter 5 focus on aspects of their etiquette that they can improve. Students will find ample room to write their answers.

- **Role-Play Scenario.** Each chapter presents a role-playing scenario for students. Directions describe how to set up the scenario, and questions lead students to observe what is wrong and what is right about how everyone acts. Space for recording answers is provided.

- **Readiness Checklist.** All chapters conclude with a Readiness Checklist to ensure that students understand all the objectives presented within the chapter. Students will find a place to check off the objectives as they learn them.
- **Journal.** At the end of this book, lined pages are provided on which students can take notes as they make their way through the program or can journal their practicum thoughts and experiences.
- **Spotlight On . . .** These features throughout the chapters highlight a variety of allied health specialties and how the practicum is important and beneficial in each area presented.

New to This Edition

This third edition includes a new full-color layout; updated, new, and expanded content; and several new features:

- New section on the right mind-set a student should have going into his or her site training
- Updated information on nontraditional interviewing, specifically phone and video interviews
- Elaboration on communicating effectively in professional relationships
- New section on communicating effectively with patient subgroups
- Overview and awareness of LinkedIn profiles
- More details on applying for jobs after the practicum
- Spotlight on Medical Assisting Certification

Acknowledgments

I would like to extend appreciation to the following reviewers for providing valuable feedback for the current and past editions of this text:

Peter F. Andrus, MD
Clinical Instructor
Albany Medical College
Albany, New York

Dominica Austin, BSN
Academic Dean
Lincoln College of Technology
Marietta, Georgia

Tricia Berry, MATL, OTR/L
Director of Clinical Placement
Kaplan University
Des Moines, Iowa

Beth Anne Buchholz, BS, CMA
Medical Assisting Department Chair
Wichita Area Technical College
Wichita, Kansas

Estelle Coffino, MPA, RRT, CPFT,
    CCMA
Associate Professor/Program
    Director
The College of Westchester
White Plains, New York

Ursula Cole, MEd, CMA, CCS-P, CHI
Medical Program Coordinator
Indiana Business College
Indianapolis, Indiana

Bernadette Cox, AAS, RMS, AHI,
    BLS Certified Instructor
Administrative and Clinic
    Instructor
Ross Medical Education Center
Flint, Michigan

Dawn Eitel, AAS, CMA
Medical Assisting Program
    Director
Kirkwood Community College
Cedar Rapids, Iowa

Cindy Garman, CMA
Medical Program Director/Director
    of Career Services
Akron Institute
Akron, Ohio

Robyn Gohsman, AAS, RMA,
    CMAS
Medical Assisting Program
    Director
Medical Careers Institute
Newport News, Virginia

Deborah E. Jacobs, RN, ENA,
    PCT
Medical Instructor
Dorsey Schools
Pontiac, Michigan

Francie Mooney, CMA (AAMA)
Faculty Medical Assisting
North Seattle College
Seattle, Washington

Lisa Nagle, BSEd, CMA
Medical Assisting Program Director
Augusta Technical Institute
Augusta, Georgia

Julie Rismiller, CMA
Clinical Externship Coordinator
Lincoln Technical Institute
Allentown, Pennsylvania

Christian G. Rivera, DC, MS
Adjunct Instructor
Florida Technical College
Deland, Florida

Janet Sesser, RMA, CMA, BS
Associate Vice President of Education
Chubb Institute
Phoenix, Arizona

Donna Stevenson, BA, LPN, CAHI
Allied Health Department Chair
Remington College
Largo, Florida

Nancy Wright, RN, BS CNOR
Instructor, College of Health Sciences
Virginia College
Birmingham, Alabama

Kim Bender, MS

The Link Between Your Education and Your Career

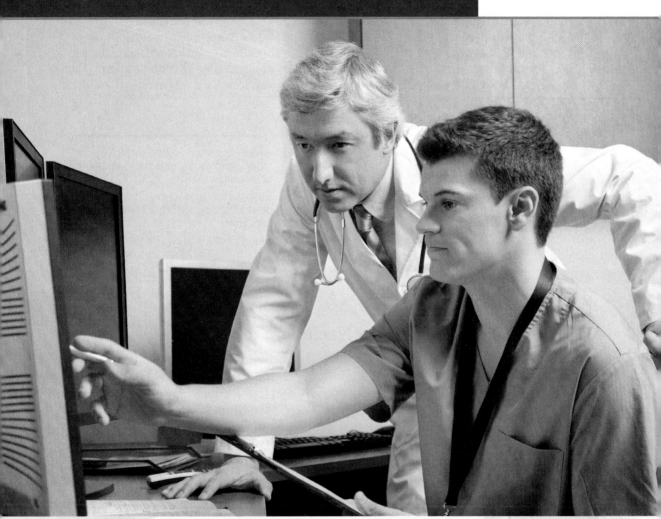

Tyler Olson/Shutterstock

The practicum provides students with valuable learning opportunities from professionals in the field of health care.

INTRODUCTION

This chapter presents basic information concerning the logic behind the concept of the practicum as an integral part of an allied health career training. To add substance and reality to this introductory concept, the chapter emphasizes several factors to remember and practice during this phase of learning. These factors include gaining real-world experience, functioning as part of an organized professional team, abiding by the major legal and ethical standards of the industry, and realizing the significance of applying such professional skills as organization, time management, and multitasking. The overall goal is to reveal how various topics and lessons from your classroom training will transfer into the real world in the practicum. The chapter concludes with Self-Prep Questions, a Role-Play Scenario, and a Readiness Checklist.

CHAPTER OBJECTIVES

- Identify the link from the classroom to the career created by the practicum.
- Identify the basic meaning of *"practicum"* and its synonymous terms.
- Describe the overall purpose of the practicum.
- Describe what it means to work as part of a health care team.
- Recall important legal and ethical considerations to be acted on during the practicum.
- Describe how organizational and time management skills are important during the practicum.
- Briefly describe multitasking.

The Importance of Your Practicum

The time to prepare has arrived. It is likely that you are in the final phases of your classroom training and are knocking on the door of your professional career in allied health. In addition to completing your classroom work, you need to take just one more step: the practicum. Many students simply accept that they will fulfill their practical phase without actually understanding the reasons or priceless benefits of doing so. The reason is fairly simple: Practicing skills in the classroom is worlds apart from the real-world medical office, clinic, outpatient center, hospital, pharmacy, or other health care setting.

The Big Transition: Student to Professional

Think of your practicum as a bridge you must cross to go from the familiar, comfortable classroom to your real-world professional career. In the classroom, a professional instructor is readily available to correct you and give you as many chances as you need to successfully acquire a certain skill or professional trait. Often, you are well acquainted with your classmates and instructors and able to learn within your comfort zone. This changes quite a bit the first day you walk through the door of your assigned training site. However, this shift is for the best, as it builds on your professional experience, and it is likely that you will discover it is valuable to you personally, too.

During the practicum, the office staff understands that you are an apprentice on the path to becoming a competent specialist in your chosen profession. While crossing this bridge, you have the experience of building your independence while realizing your interdependence within a team, further developing your practical skills, and developing your professionalism in many other ways. Take advantage of the advice and constructive criticism that professionals offer you in this text—absorbing their insights will contribute greatly to your store of knowledge, and as you read you will become more aware of the many benefits of this phase of learning.

What Is Meant by *Practicum*?

The word *practicum* is interchangeable with the terms *externship*, *practical experience*, *clinical rotation*, and *internship*, among others. All these terms directly capture the concept of students practicing clinical or other specialized practical skills in a professionally supervised, off-campus, real-world setting as part of a program of study. Although an array of allied health specialties exists, each with its own unique set of required achievements for students in training, the common purpose of the practical experience among these professions is to successfully apply relevant skills and knowledge in a professional setting. All clinically trained students must complete a practicum, and even many administratively focused students are required to do so as well.

Applying Your Skills and Knowledge

Practicing your clinical and other practical skills is one of the most important objectives you must achieve. Some students assume they will have the opportunity to acquire (rather than refine) their skills while practicing at the practicum site. Although some sites may provide time and an available staff member to assist trainees in mastering a certain skill, most office managers and facility supervisors expect that the student has already mastered most necessary skills practiced in the classroom. For example, determining a patient's blood pressure manually is a skill that requires concentration, accuracy, and precision. It is a skill that must be learned through repetitious practice over time. It is expected that you are already competent in this particular skill if you are a medical assistant (MA); you should be comfortable, efficient, and correct when performing it. Busy health care facilities typically allow no time to relearn skills that were practiced and tested in the classroom.

The overall purpose of your practicum, if clinically focused, is to apply the skills acquired in the classroom to a real-world setting where patients are sick, moody, depressed, agitated, or impatient with the prolonged process of checking in to see their providers. If your practicum is, for example, in the realm of insurance and billing or health information, the general purpose will be to exercise your efficiency and accuracy in handling claims, applying diagnosis and procedure codes, verifying insurance, discussing account information with patients and payers, functioning within the team, and so on, all in a fast-paced setting where managers are concerned with timely and accurate reimbursement. During a practicum in pharmacy technology, students must focus on several areas, such as customer service, assisting in insurance verification, working within a team of one or more pharmacists and other technicians, and practicing proper handling and dispensing of drugs.

Professionalism: The Highest Calling

In all practical training-site programs, facility managers, doctors, pharmacists, and other health care professionals expect utmost professionalism from student-trainees. Classroom time generally does not provide the opportunity to polish the more professional and personal side of working within the industry, and the practicum experience is extremely valuable for working on these skills. For the benefit of all student readers, it is noted here that most practicum failures or below-average outcomes are generally because of lack of professionalism. In other words, your effort to maintain your professionalism is usually the factor that determines the success or failure of your practicum. Therefore, focus throughout your pre-practicum classroom study on developing and refining your professional attributes for the sake of your off-site practical training and your soon-to-follow career. Various aspects of how student-trainees' level of professionalism affects their practicum (and future career) are discussed throughout this text.

Becoming Part of the Health Care Team

In any allied health practicum, in addition to serving patient needs in the ways that are unique to your given specialty, you will be practicing the art of participating as an active and vital member of an important health care team. This also entails developing skills that are unattainable solely from classroom experience. Today's medical office teams are expected to be efficient, but that efficiency must not compromise the effectiveness or quality of care provided to patients.

Typically, an average medical office staff might include the following:

- Front desk/administrative personnel (e.g., handling reception, appointments, faxes and phones, patient sign-in)
- Billing and insurance representatives
- Patient records specialists
- Administrator or office manager
- Specialized technicians (X-ray, lab/phlebotomy, etc.)
- Medical assistant(s)
- Nurse(s)

- Nurse practitioner(s) (NP)
- Physician assistant(s) (PA)
- Physician(s)

In particular, the MA serves as an important link between both front and back offices. Likewise, those students practicing in the specialty of administrative office, as well as billing and coding, must blend into a functioning team, effectively contributing to the tasks at hand so that the complete order and functioning of the facility are maintained. The team aspect is also a significant factor in the efficiency of pharmacies, dental offices, surgery centers, and so on. It is also important to practice the large-scale team concept that spans various facilities or organizations, while recognizing the interdependency among all areas of patient service necessary for the overall delivery of health care. An example of this large-scale, multifacility teamwork is the communication that takes place between a medical practice's MA or nurse and the pharmacist or pharmacy technician when a prescription is ordered or called in for a patient.

The practicum provides you a golden opportunity to become an integral part of this large-scale team, in whatever specialization you practice, proving to yourself and other professionals that you are a valuable asset. This learning experience is tremendously beneficial and helps you develop professional skills that can be used in future career placement and advancement. The practicum is likely to be the first place where your education can be integrated as you practice in close association with other team members.

Spotlight on Medical Assisting: Teamwork Experience During the Practicum

Members of office/facility-based health care teams as well as teams or networks of providers rely on MAs for a wide variety of essential tasks in the ongoing cycle of patient care. MAs often serve to connect front and back office tasks in traditional medical office settings. In addition, they serve as the point of contact for patients' health-related phone calls and communicate with nurses and doctors on behalf of patients. Reaching beyond the confines of their workplace, they also serve as the point of contact for their office with outside providers, specialists, labs, pharmacies, and so on. MA student-trainees can catch a realistic glimpse of this hingelike role during the practicum and will perhaps be able to experience how so many individuals from all areas of health care truly rely on their skills and coordination to provide effective patient care.

Gaining Experience with Legal and Ethical Considerations

Do you recall the medical law and ethics topics emphasized in your program of study? Do you remember the importance of professional liability issues,

Health Information Portability and Accountability Act (HIPAA) compliance, patient confidentiality, the potential use of a patient's chart as a legal document, and such? Well, here it is, once again, in *real-world* application. Adhering to professional standards in these areas is extremely important. Directly applicable to your duties as an MA or other allied health professional, you will communicate constantly in person (face-to-face), over the phone, via fax, as well as through e-mail, primarily regarding patients and their ailments, health history, prescriptions, lab work and diagnostic testing, billing and insurance, office and facility issues, and so on. You must use professional discretion in how and where you communicate patient information to your co-workers. Basic behaviors you will need to practice are speaking softly and privately to your patients and customers, keeping medical charts closed when you are not making notes in them, and speaking softly over the phone if you are communicating with a patient or about a patient. Also, keep in mind the significance of every piece of information you record in a patient's file or chart—documentation must be accurate because at any time any patient chart can be subpoenaed as a legal document for court proceedings. Unfortunately, substantial time is typically unavailable in the classroom setting for elaborate role-playing of these necessary applications. Practicing according to the applicable legal and ethical standards of your discipline is not only a requirement but also a critical component of your overall qualification to work successfully as an allied health professional.

Organization and Time Management Applications

Organization and time management are other professional skills you will build on during the practicum. These are learned to some extent while attending class, managing your homework and projects, and studying for comprehensive course exams. Perhaps you have had the opportunity to practice these skills in your previous employment endeavors. However, managing patients and helping maintain order in the office are, again, specific and necessary skills you can learn only by experience.

Chart or document organization, preparing patient rooms, and clinical and administrative tasks are major areas in which you must demonstrate punctuality. Your performance should demonstrate quality work at or above the professional standard of care and practice, not merely a haphazard effort to keep pace. You must apply quality and correctness in your work as much as efficiency. You cannot afford to make mistakes when assessing vital signs, recording information in patient charts, or communicating information verbally to other medical office staff or to representatives in other facilities, always keeping in mind the legal aspects of the patient medical record.

Regardless of your area of practice, you will learn to manage several different and possibly unrelated responsibilities in a given period of time (i.e., to multitask). *Multitasking* is increasingly necessary in today's workplace, and grasping how to implement it will build the list of professional skills you develop while on practicum. Everyone working in your facility will have to manage his or her time, too. Learning how to effectively manage your time to meet the expected level of productivity will provide you with another important, experience-based skill you will need for a successful allied health career.

HIGHLIGHT

TIPS FROM PROFESSIONALS

There exists much value in the practicum, and students should make the most of their opportunity. Those who go into their practical training with excitement and anticipation, a professional mindset and positive attitude are typically the ones who excel. I have hired some of the students our office has hosted for practical training; the best candidates demonstrate proficient skill level matched by professional qualities and a desirable mindset.

Some recommendations to students for the practicum are, first and foremost, take your practicum seriously, and treat it like you would a professional job. Keep a positive attitude and be proactive in your learning. Be responsible and ready to learn each day of your training, simply give your best effort.

–Owner and President (medical billing company)

Conclusion

Many benefits and necessary considerations beyond those mentioned in this chapter are worth looking forward to, as you will learn in later chapters. However, this chapter addresses some of the foremost reasons why your practicum is a necessary part of your comprehensive education and training as a medical assistant, health information technician, office assistant, pharmacy technician, dental hygienist, or other allied health professional. If the practicum will be your first experience in any health care setting, the time you spend is even more valuable and important to you in your quest to enter the challenging yet rewarding industry of allied health.

Self-Prep Questions

1. What do you believe you personally have to gain from your practicum?

_____

_____

_____

_____

_____

2. List at least five important purposes for completing the practicum.

_____

_____

_____

_____

3. Find out, write down, and remember the number of hours you are expected to complete. How many hours are required of you on a daily or weekly basis? If you are in a program with clinical rotations through different practice areas, write down your scheduled hour requirements for each rotation.

_____

_____

_____

_____

_____

4. What are at least three basic skills you can practice to ensure patient confidentiality?

_____

_____

_____

_____

_____

5. Why is accuracy of documentation in patient charts so important?

_____

_____

_____

_____

Role-Play Scenario

Three individuals are needed for this scenario: the student-trainee, the receptionist, and the office manager. Suppose it is your first day of the practicum. You walk into the medical office and tell the receptionist you are there to begin your practicum and that you need to meet with Patty, the office manager, first. The receptionist locates Patty and informs her that you have arrived for your first day of training. Role-play the scenario in which Patty comes to greet you, gives you an office overview and tour, and introduces you to the staff members. As Patty is talking with you and walking you through the office, demonstrate your overall idea of professionalism. To start, first consider some major aspects that contribute to professionalism. (For example, a few ways to show professionalism might be through your attentiveness to what Patty says, paying attention/listening so that you can ask appropriate questions, and appearing interested and ready to learn and work.)

1. How will you present yourself professionally to give a good first impression? Consider your dress and appearance, mannerisms, communication tactics, and so on.

_____

_____

_____

_____

_____

2. Because you do not yet know much about this office and how it functions, what are some intelligent questions you can ask Patty as she is introducing you to the office setting and staff? (Keep in mind that these types of questions demonstrate your overall interest in the profession and your desire to learn.)

_____

_____

_____

_____

_____

3. After this introduction to the facility and tour, how would you express to Patty some of what you are interested in learning so that she can help you work toward your goals?

_____

_____

_____

_____

_____

Readiness Checklist

_____ I understand why the practicum is required of health care professionals.

_____ I understand the differences between classroom learning and the experiential learning that I will complete during the practicum.

_____ I understand what is meant by working as part of a professional team.

_____ I understand the importance of patient confidentiality and of measures such as HIPAA that ensure it is maintained.

_____ I know where I can find resources that will review the standard of care and code of ethics regarding my practice as a medical assistant or other allied health professional.

_____ I understand that I am to be discreet in communicating patient information.

_____ I understand the ways in which my organization, time management, and multitasking skills will be exercised during my practicum.

Meeting and Exceeding Expectations

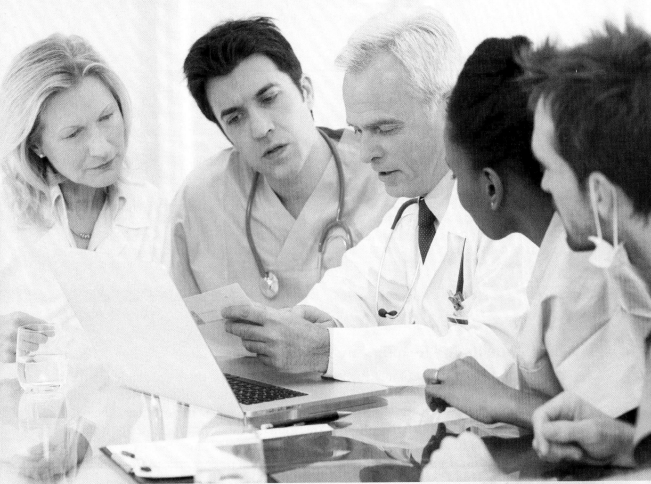

Rido/Fotolia

Site supervisors expect students to take a proactive and professional approach in learning during the practicum.

INTRODUCTION

This chapter presents various expectations that all future student-trainees should heed in advance of their practicum. First, various common college, school, and departmental requirements are presented, followed by the expectations that practicum site managers and trainers have of students. This foreknowledge will help students realize the importance of completing all documentation and other academic or school requirements on time, as well as understanding the minimum expectations held by the professionals providing the on-site training. The chapter concludes with Self-Prep Questions, a Role-Play Scenario, and a Readiness Checklist.

CHAPTER OBJECTIVES

- Identify the two parties to whom the student-trainee is responsible.
- Recognize student-trainee health documentation that may be required before the practicum.
- Identify the requirements typically imposed by career/professional services departments within colleges and career training schools.
- Understand the benefits of timely submission of all required pre-practicum paperwork and documentation.
- Identify the reasons why students should always present to their practicum site with a resumé.

- Explain the typical process of submitting completed site hours to the school for practicum course attendance.
- Describe how performance is linked to the final course grade.
- Identify miscellaneous requirements commonly imposed by schools.
- Describe the expected manner for handling communication issues regarding tardiness to or absence from the practicum site.
- Identify the typical expectations of the practicum site supervisor and staff/trainers concerning student-trainees.

Students Are Responsible to Two Parties

In general, students must fulfill the expectations of their academic institution as well as their practicum site supervisors and trainers. Meeting and exceeding the expectations of both parties are of equal importance. The best action students can take is to ask questions and be sure to have a thorough understanding of these expectations before the practicum begins. Typically, a practicum coordinator or other faculty member/instructor (perhaps with a differing title) from your school will be completely responsible for overseeing the practicum phase. This person will also be the school's point of contact for the site supervisor.

Expectations of the Academic Institution and Faculty

In most cases, pre-practicum requirements must be met first. These normally include a physical exam, a tuberculosis (TB) test, immunizations (especially for participation in a clinical practicum), proof of student liability insurance (many schools provide this for their students), resumé and cover letter completion, and other professional and health requirements such as a cardio-pulmonary resuscitation (CPR) or basic life support (BLS) certification and a practical skills competency check. Submitting timesheets or records of hours as specified, maintaining contact with the faculty coordinator, and putting forth effort to learn are required throughout the practicum.

Completing all practicum requirements on time is extremely important. In addition to expected academic consequences, delays in beginning and completing the practicum can have financial consequences (especially for those students receiving federal financial aid).

Each individual school has its own specific procedures and documentation requirements. The following subsections pertain to students' typical responsibilities in relation to their academic institution and cover a wide variety of requirements likely to be imposed by most schools:

- Health documentation requirements
- Student practice liability insurance
- Career services department requirements
- Submission of timesheet/record of practicum site hours
- The effort expended
- Additional requirements

HEALTH DOCUMENTATION REQUIREMENTS

For clinically oriented practicum programs, almost every school stipulates a set of health/medical requirements and forms that students must complete before the practicum start date. These vary by school but generally involve a comprehensive physical exam along with certain immunizations/vaccinations and TB testing. Whatever the requirements are at the practicum site, you must complete and submit this paperwork on time. The school will not allow students to participate in the practicum without the required documentation. This involves advanced planning on your part, considering that you will probably have to wait for a medical appointment to fulfill these requirements.

You should locate or obtain immunization records early in this process. This documentation is not always kept with current personal health records and may require an extensive search, such as contacting a former family doctor or pediatrician for copies.

While completing these health requirements and before submitting them to your school, confirm that all information is legible and that all dates and signatures are visible. These documents (or copies of them) will be filed in your official student record.

Failure to supply this documentation will undoubtedly prevent you from beginning your practicum, maintaining your status as a student-trainee, and attending classes.

STUDENT PRACTICE LIABILITY INSURANCE

Another required item for your practicum, which either will be your responsibility or will be provided by your school, is student professional liability insurance. Some schools subscribe to insurers providing coverage for all students in specified programs. However, some schools require students to purchase student professional liability insurance before their practicum. If you do not know how this applies to you, it is best to ask your faculty adviser or program director about the requirements. Although this is typically required and covered by the school, many practicum site managers will not allow a student to begin the practicum without proof of this insurance. Although this is the combined responsibility of both you and your school, it is only mentioned in this section to avoid repetitiveness.

CAREER SERVICES DEPARTMENT REQUIREMENTS

Many colleges, especially those with a career services/resources department, require students to complete a resumé, cover letter, and exit interview before graduating. These requirements may be due early when programs provide a practicum at the conclusion of the program. Meeting your institution's due dates for graduation requirements ensures that you will gain at least three benefits: First, completing all paperwork ensures that you will not have any setbacks when it comes to receiving your official graduate status and diploma or degree; second, your career/employment services director/representative will have extra time to help you refine your resumé and begin assisting you in your job search; and third, you will not have any documentation setbacks that would prevent you from beginning the practicum on time. Beginning the practicum late will likely delay your graduation date, and it may affect your practicum course grade.

As noted, the resumé is an important document at this time. It is to your benefit to take your completed, professional resumé to the practicum site. For starters, it is the professional thing to do. This practicum could be your first point of entry into the health care industry, and therefore, you should make your best first impression, even though technically you are still a student. Your resumé is useful in delineating previous jobs, responsibilities, and education, especially the allied health education you have been pursuing in recent months or years. Be sure to include any volunteer work, especially if it involves helping in a patient care setting of any sort. A detailed discussion of building an effective resumé is presented in Chapter 11 of this text.

SUBMISSION OF TIMESHEET OR RECORD OF PRACTICUM SITE HOURS

Timesheets or timecards for recording your practicum hours can be handled in various ways. These may be given to you, or they may be distributed to your practicum site supervisor directly by the program faculty. If they are in your possession, be sure to keep them in a safe place. Once you officially begin the practicum, ask your supervisor if there is a safe place in the office where you may store them. Slightly different procedures are imposed by different schools, but the main concept is that a clear and verifiable record of the hours you were present and participating at the site must be maintained. Typically, your hours will not be recognized as officially complete by your college until a signature or verbal verification of the supervisor, or both, is obtained by the school's practicum program coordinator. This is very important because the hours completed and submitted translate directly to your attendance record. It is to your benefit to keep a photocopy or electronic copy of these records, with signatures, as you would (and will) for an actual job. You may be instructed to electronically submit or fax documentation of your completed hours each week or so, or you may be required to submit them in person to your school practicum coordinator.

Both your practicum coordinator and your site supervisor will expect you to handle the submission of your completed site hours documentation professionally; this includes being punctual, honest, and following appropriate procedures.

Unfortunately, some students are tempted to exaggerate a few hours here and there on their timesheet; however, anyone who has tried this has usually been caught and, when caught, has always been penalized. Because of the communication between the school's liaison or coordinator to the practicum site and the staff at the site, false time credits are easily detectable. All students in training should refrain from this type of dishonest behavior as it inevitably sets the stage for failure or some other negative consequence. It is also important to recognize that your practicum site supervisor is *not* the person ultimately responsible for submitting your record of hours, unless this is arranged between your school and the site supervisor.

Remember: Abiding by the procedures related to timekeeping will help you to develop your abilities to be a responsible and accountable professional.

THE EFFORT EXPENDED

You will, of course, be expected to perform your best and learn as you gain experience. Toward the end of your practical experience, your site supervisor and a faculty member from your school, or both, will evaluate you. Your college may request several periodic evaluations or just one on completion of your practicum. Most colleges will determine your overall practicum course grade largely based on how your supervisor rates your performance in these evaluations. Generally, a comprehensive evaluation form for a medical assisting practicum includes specific competencies in the categories of clinical, practical, and administrative duties, as well as attributes of professionalism that you did or did not demonstrate while practicing. Similar organization applies to almost every allied health specialty. For example, administrative, professional, and practical skills are specified on evaluation forms for fields such as medical billing and coding, health information, pharmacy technology, dental hygiene, and so on. Knowing this, you probably will conclude that your practicum should be taken seriously and demands the professionalism of an actual job. If possible, request from your program faculty a sample copy of the evaluation form by which your performance will be rated. Use this form for reference before and throughout your practicum experience. You can use the evaluation as a pre-practicum preparation tool to identify technical skills or competencies for which you feel you need extra practice or review before going to practice in the field. Chapter 9 contains more information concerning how you will be evaluated, along with a few sample evaluation forms.

ADDITIONAL REQUIREMENTS

Before the practicum, your school may have some additional requirements. For example, the individual departments within your school may have to sign certain paperwork to demonstrate that you have met their respective requirements for graduation. It is likely that you will have to be trained in CPR, first aid, and/or BLS before the practicum, with your valid certification card serving as proof of completion. Once you have fulfilled this requirement and received a certification card, be sure to submit a copy for your student file and to include the certification and effective date on your resumé.

You also may be required to provide a written or signed verification from your clinical instructor(s)/faculty to indicate that you have mastered all skill areas relevant to your program. This is particularly important for medical assistants and other clinically trained students attempting to complete an accredited program. Many schools have an established practical skills test that students must pass to prove their competency before the practicum. Even if this is not a stipulated requirement at your school or college, you should still seek verification by your instructors, for your own benefit, that you are completely competent in all skills. In addition, it may be required that student-trainees undergo a drug test, a background check, or both before the practicum. This requirement can be imposed by either your school or the training site.

Communication with your supervising faculty or practicum coordinator on a regular basis is vital. If you have any days during which you are ill or have a valid excuse for arriving late to the site, you must call your site supervisor or at least communicate with a staff member regarding the issue; additionally, you must speak to or at least leave a message for your school's coordinator concerning the situation. It is imperative to inform both your coordinator and site manager of this situation at the same time. Because timeliness is important, contact the site supervisor as soon as possible, just as you would for an actual job. If the practicum site was your employer and you failed to report your absence with a timely phone call, you might not have that job by day's end. Students have been dismissed from their practicum sites for not arriving as scheduled and failing to make contact with a phone call.

On the first day of your practicum, ask your site supervisor what additional steps are required beyond these basic notification procedures in case you are late or unable to attend. Be sure to keep the appropriate contact information readily available.

You are expected to take responsibility and communicate appropriately in all such cases. The communication skills you exhibit are a significant indicator of your overall level of professionalism.

In summary, before your practicum start date, you should verify with your practicum program coordinator that everything required of you is officially completed. If you find yourself lagging in doing this, realize that finalizing these requirements on time will save you the time and stress it takes to get them done at the last minute.

Expectations of the Practicum Site Staff and Trainers

The following points pertaining to general expectations of the professionals working on site with students during the practicum are discussed throughout the following subsections.

- The right attitude
- Punctuality and effective communication
- Proactive learning
- Adaptability in the workplace
- Willingness to cross-train
- Recognition of protective measures for health care workers

THE RIGHT ATTITUDE

Your success in the practicum will largely depend on your attitude. Although this text covers more on "attitudes" in Chapter 4, this section will address one major attitude factor that must be considered up front—and remembered. It is imperative that the mindset going into your site training is that you (or any other student) are *not* doing the hosting site a favor, or providing free labor, by attending the site as scheduled and working. It is quite the opposite: The site staff is doing you a favor. The site manager/trainers expect that you understand this, and whether you do or do not is reflected by your attitude. Keep in mind that you are a still a student, without yet having attained professional status in your chosen field. All professionals (in any career field) begin in some type or preceptorship or training, even if their academic program does not require a practicum per se. In reality, you want to be as well trained, aware, and prepared as possible *before* you enter a paid, professional position where the expectations are much higher. Unfortunately, it is typical that the small handful of students embarking on their practicum while holding the wrong view (that they are doing the site a favor) end up falling short in their performance—their mindset simply is not in the right place, and they feel they need not put in the effort or that they are receiving any benefit. When a site agrees to host you, the student, to train you and provide you so many hours of real-world experience (which are required of you in order to graduate), this is something for which to be grateful and to be seen as an opportunity.

Many benefits can be realized through the practicum experience, which are discussed in detail in Chapter 8. Therefore, be sure to make any needed adjustments in your perception of the practicum before beginning.

PUNCTUALITY AND EFFECTIVE COMMUNICATION

When physician offices or other medical facilities agree to provide a training atmosphere for new allied health workers, they agree to it with several expectations of you, the student. Your trainers will expect you to arrive as scheduled (on time) and ready to train, attending to the full shift productively with the intent to work and learn. Your supervisor or trainer expects you to be as professional as the rest of the staff. One expectation is that, for the short term of your practicum, there should be no absences or tardiness issues. Not arriving as scheduled and being late convey lack of professionalism and work ethic. If there is an absence, normal professional protocol, as described previously in this chapter, should be followed. Make telephone contact ahead of time; do not waltz through the door late, even if you are late only by five minutes, without a phone call, and then expect no consequences. Even if your site seems to be a friendly and comfortable environment, where being late may not seem detrimental to daily operations, somebody will always take notice, especially if these events are habitual throughout your practicum.

HIGHLIGHT

TIPS FROM PROFESSIONALS

My advice to students is to take your practical training seriously, adhering to all the professional traits you would make sure to show in a professional job role. Imagine you are being observed and assessed for your suitability for an upcoming position with the office/site…this often happens! In this case you would want to make known your punctuality, responsibility, communication skills, readiness and trainability. Make the most of it!

–Administrative Coordinator (pediatrics office)

PROACTIVE LEARNING

Two specific areas regarding the expectation that you must "work your full shift productively with intent to learn" merit further explanation. First, the word *full* describing *shift* means that leaving earlier than scheduled is unacceptable, except in case of a true emergency. As always, somebody will observe your actions. The other key term is *productively*. While at the practicum site, you are expected, at the very least, to be proactive in your learning and take initiative. To learn proactively, you must participate by taking notes, keeping a journal, asking questions, volunteering, and so on, even during any slow times of day. Those training you will see this as professional on your part; it shows them that you are motivated, interested in your field of study, and trainable. Your diligence to learn proactively may be a heavily weighted factor in a supervisor's decision to hire you. Once you are familiar with the workings of the facility to which you are assigned, you should exhibit initiative in keeping up the pace. At no time of the day should you be doing nothing. Never sit around and wait to be told what to do, and never use slow times to catch up on your nonpracticum business, like spending time on your phone, listening to personal voice mail, returning phone calls, texting, e-mailing, or engaging in other personal tasks. At such times, ask what you can do to help in another area of the office, even if it is cleaning up or reorganizing the office desk or patient waiting area. Your initiative will impress managers and potential employers because it shows that you work with a caring and positive attitude.

ADAPTABILITY IN THE WORKPLACE

Another professional skill that site staff will expect you to demonstrate is *adaptability*. How easily can you adapt to change? If a new manager takes over your site during your practicum, and your duties are suddenly more varied than before, can you handle it? Furthermore, can you handle it *professionally*? What if new software for the office is implemented while you are on your practicum, once you just finished learning the prior system? What if another employee is on leave for a week because of illness or surgery and the manager asks you to come in an hour earlier each day of that week to help carry the workload? Most people would agree that these tasks are doable. However, changes may occur at an unexpected or inopportune time, and with this may come some level of inconvenience to you, depending on the nature of the change. Nonetheless, if you must face the challenge of change, the professional way to handle it is to willingly cooperate with the rest of the team. It is even more important to do so without complaining, while exhibiting a positive attitude and professionalism. If you experience a change at your site and experience difficulty in learning or adapting to the new task or procedure—despite your most honest effort to catch on—it is important to inform your site supervisor or a staff member so that further training can be arranged for you. Change in the workplace is inevitable—therefore, exercising your flexibility in this area during the practicum, if necessary, will benefit you.

HIGHLIGHT

TIPS FROM PROFESSIONALS

A good way to approach your site training is to do the same as you would to prepare for a test. Be sure to bring a notebook each day and make notes on all you are learning, and reinforce your learning by revisiting those notes and reflecting on your experiences.

–Medical Assistant (Cardiology office)

WILLINGNESS TO CROSS-TRAIN

Even if you have been educated in only one concentration or discipline, your site manager will likely have a system of cross-training prepared for you. Medical assistants, especially, should expect to take part in cross-training during the practicum. Whatever the case, you must be prepared to accept the breadth of the training provided to you. For example, you may be preparing for a practicum in medical assisting and your favorite tasks are to perform phlebotomies and administer injections; however, the site manager is planning for you to complete a schedule of mornings working one-on-one with patients in the back office and performing certain clinical tasks, then spending afternoons assisting and learning such front office tasks as scheduling, filing insurance claims, ordering labs, and prescriptions. Although students typically prefer certain tasks to others, your training program must be comprehensive, and it is to your benefit to gladly receive the training offered in all areas. For medical assistants engaging in the practicum under the American Association of Medical Assistants (AAMA) regulations, specific division of front and back office experience is a requirement. For future employment purposes, you will be able to document this cross-training experience, if applicable, on your post-practicum resumé. The training staff also expects you to be willing to learn in this way.

Another benefit of cross-training during your practicum is that you will understand how your specific tasks and responsibilities contribute to the overall functioning of the practicum site. Gaining this perspective will help you professionally because your understanding will lead to increased effectiveness in your specialty.

RECOGNITION OF PROTECTIVE MEASURES FOR HEALTH CARE WORKERS

For clinically trained student-trainees, the site supervisor will likely assume that you are well aware of the Bloodborne Pathogens Standard of the Occupational Safety and Health Administration (OSHA) as well as the Universal Precautions for Preventing Transmission of Bloodborne Infections of the Centers for Disease Control and Prevention (CDC). If you feel you do not know or have forgotten any of the specifics related to these standards, you must master them before your practicum. Your practicum site will have a way for you to access this information. However, do not arrive at your site without a general knowledge of what the regulations cover and why they exist. In addition, be sure you remember the guidelines covering the use of personal protective equipment (PPE).

Obviously, these regulations and guidelines are more applicable in some facilities than in others; for instance, in an outpatient surgical center or dental specialty facility, these would be referenced much more often than they would in a primary care office, a claims processing office, or a retail pharmacy. Also, some professionals will not need to apply/practice these guidelines if their particular work within the facility does not call for adherence to them; for instance, neither the human resources (HR) office employees of a large medical group or hospital nor the business manager of an outpatient surgical center would be in a position in their line of work to regularly follow the Bloodborne Pathogens Standard, the Universal Precautions, or the use of

PPE. By the time you begin your practicum, you should know the extent to which these guidelines apply to your specific function within allied health.

Realistic Expectations Concerning the Site

Going into the practicum, students generally have a mental picture of how their experience will work, what the atmosphere and the employees will be like, what they will be able to learn, and what experience they will gain. Students should generally expect that their site supervisor will train them and assign them tasks aligned with those of current staff members within the same specialty. However, it is important for students to realize that each site, although working with colleges to provide practical experience opportunities to students, is still its own entity and has its own policies, procedures, processes, and expectations. Therefore, it is important for students to be flexible and understand that they are subject to the site's methods and management during the practicum.

The following are some examples of what students should expect upon starting their practicum at their site:

- The site will create its own method for training students based on how and where the student will best fit in. This will include consideration of when the appropriate trainer is available for the areas to be covered. This can also be based on the need for help in a certain area at a certain time, or on a plan to start with a certain task and gradually build up to more complex tasks and responsibilities over time.
- The site manager may stipulate tasks or responsibilities that students are not allowed to handle because of the policies of the facility. For example, allied health students in hospital settings often are not allowed to access or work directly with patient medical records because of more stringent corporate policies on patient confidentiality. Medical offices are often more flexible with students in this regard provided the student proves competent in the HIPAA law. Similar limitations may also exist for answering incoming phone calls and working with patient accounts.
- The site supervisor may ask the student to adopt a certain dress code that is in alignment with that of the regular staff, may purposely request the student to present differently, or may give the student general attire guidelines that allow some flexibility.

Going Above and Beyond

You can go above and beyond all expectations by preparing yourself for the career you hope to establish after the practicum. Joining a professional organization and preparing yourself for certification can help demonstrate your commitment to the allied health field.

Join a Professional Organization as a Student Member

While completing your coursework, apply for student membership in a professional organization for your chosen field. You can document this membership on your resumé, and this will communicate to the health care community that you are dedicated to becoming a fully qualified professional. It shows your site supervisor and potential employers that you have joined your peers in a professional association and are being exposed through that organization to the most recent standards, advancements, and ethical requirements in the field.

Prepare Early for Registration and Certification in Your Profession

Become certified or registered in your profession as soon as you are able once all prerequisites for the certification are met. Most certifying entities require the completion of and graduation from an accredited program of study before exam-based certification. Generally, applications to sit for such exams are to be submitted well in advance of the actual test date. Planning ahead is necessary if you wish to become professionally credentialed within a reasonable period after graduation. Your allied health department faculty should be able to direct you to the appropriate point of contact for obtaining application materials, or your school may deal directly with some of these organizations to provide on-site testing. Once you have obtained the registration materials, carefully consider the test date for which you will be eligible, and take note of the application due date and any additional documentation requirements for completion of your application. For example, some of the organizations require references or letters of recommendation, along with your basic application form. Make note of the registration fee for the exam, as payment must be submitted with your application for it to be processed. (See Appendix: Selected Allied-Health Certification and Credentialing Resources at the end of this text for a listing of allied health professional organizations, the certification/registration each awards, and Web site information.)

Spotlight on Medical Billing and Coding: Student Membership with the AAPC

Medical billing and coding students have the opportunity to join the American Academy of Professional Coders (AAPC) with a student-level membership. By joining, they become introduced to the real world of billing and coding on the national level; gain access to events, seminars/webinars, and local chapter meetings; can search the database of billing and coding jobs; and can develop networking opportunities. Establishing membership in the professional organization representing this field gives students a nationally recognizable affiliation with the profession, and it shows the billing/coding student's intention to follow through with his or her program of study leading to at least one of the AAPC's nationally recognized certifications.

Once students complete their education and practicum, and become AAPC certified, they become qualified to enjoy the benefits of professional-level membership. A few perks included with this are insight from industry leaders, networking with affiliated professionals, savings on AAPC products, professional webinars, local meeting events, and more.

Conclusion

Aligning yourself with the expectations discussed in this chapter will ensure success with regard to both your dealings with your faculty coordinator and your practicum site supervisor(s). Maintain a steady focus in these areas. It is possible for the supervising staff member or manager to dismiss you from the practicum position because of professional inadequacies; it has happened to students before, but fortunately it is easily preventable. Many more professional attributes that site managers, staff trainers, and physicians expect are described throughout the remainder of this text. Continue to use this guide to evaluate yourself before the practicum so that you are well prepared for a positive and productive experience.

Self-Prep Questions

1. Do you have a particular interest regarding the medical specialty or type of facility in which you would like to work? Write down your interests and communicate them to your practicum program coordinator in advance of your practicum. Also communicate your interests to your school's career services staff.

_____

_____

_____

_____

_____

2. Acquire or make a list of your school's health (and any other) requirements that must be complete before the practicum. How far in advance must documentation be submitted?

_____

_____

_____

_____

_____

3. Write down the contact information for your practicum program coordinator, school, and medical/health instructors. Include fax number(s).

_____

_____

_____

_____

_____

4. How will your attendance and hours be monitored by your institution? What specific responsibilities are yours concerning submission of your documented site hours?

_____

_____

_____

_____

_____

5. Make a list of any skills you need to practice more. Be sure to communicate these needs to your faculty/instructors at an appropriate time before the practicum.

_____

_____

_____

_____

_____

6. Recall a situation in class, at a job, or elsewhere in which you had to quickly adapt to a new way of doing things. If you cannot recall one of your own personal experiences, create a hypothetical medical office scenario that includes a significant change and explain how you, the student-trainee, should adapt.

_____

_____

_____

_____

7. What is the name of the professional organization designated for your allied health specialty? Visit the organization's Web site. Are student memberships available? Review the general process for membership.

_____

_____

_____

_____

_____

Role-Play Scenario

Two or more individuals are needed for this scenario. Suppose the practicum program coordinator (one of the individuals) is presenting the pre-practicum requirements of your school to a group of students beginning the practicum in the near future. (If manageable, the entire class can participate as the "group" of students.) The practicum program coordinator should review all school requirements for this group with basic instructions. The group/audience (the other one or more individuals) must each ask at least two questions on different topics or requirements presented by the acting practicum program coordinator. Members of the group/audience should ask questions that test the knowledge of the practicum program coordinator, and the coordinator should ask questions and request solutions of group members regarding, for example, how to follow basic procedures, resolve problematic situations, or compile pre-practicum documents and other requirements. This exercise is intended to help participating individuals to gain a better understanding of their school's specific practicum requirements. It is most effective to perform this scenario after a thorough overview of the school's practical experience program has been delivered by faculty to students.

1. What are the main topics the practicum program coordinator would need to cover for the presentation, based on your school's practicum requirements?

_____

_____

_____

_____

_____

2. What are some details concerning some of the points made that the group can ask questions about?

_____

_____

_____

_____

_____

3. What timeframes and deadlines of importance are established for your upcoming practicum?

_____

_____

_____

_____

4. How can the practicum program coordinator make sure that the group has a thorough understanding of the requirements?

_____

_____

_____

_____

_____

Readiness Checklist

_____ I know what documentation is required of my institution's program before beginning the practicum.

_____ I know the timeframe and due dates I must meet to accomplish timely submission of these requirements.

_____ I am aware of the issue with student liability insurance, and I know whether I am responsible for this or whether my school provides appropriate coverage.

_____ I understand how to document and submit my record of attendance and hours worked at the practicum site, and I understand the consequences of not following the appropriate procedures.

_____ I understand my program's method of evaluating my performance throughout the practicum.

_____ I have received verification by my classroom and lab instructors that I am competent in my technical skills and knowledge.

_____ I understand the importance of appropriate communication with my faculty or practicum program coordinator and with my site staff trainers.

_____ I understand the minimum expectations of the practicum site managers and trainers who agree to train me at their facility.

_____ I understand that my absences and/or tardiness should be nonexistent unless an emergency is pending. If I must be absent or late, I understand the typical professional protocol for communicating this to my site supervisor.

_____ I understand that I am expected to work my full scheduled shift and to do so productively.

_____ I have identified what it means to adapt professionally to change when necessary.

_____ I understand that rather than repeating my favorite skills during my practicum, I may be assigned to learn the tasks of other areas in the office or facility. It is evident to me why this cross-training may be expected and also why it works to my advantage.

_____ I have read and understood the content of OSHA's Bloodborne Pathogens Standard and the CDC's Universal Precautions.

_____ I understand that I should expect my site supervisor to train me adequately within the scope of the site's normal daily policies and procedures, and that there is variation among training facilities in how the practicum is administered.

_____ I understand the benefits of joining a professional organization as a student member.

3 Practicum Site Placement Interviews

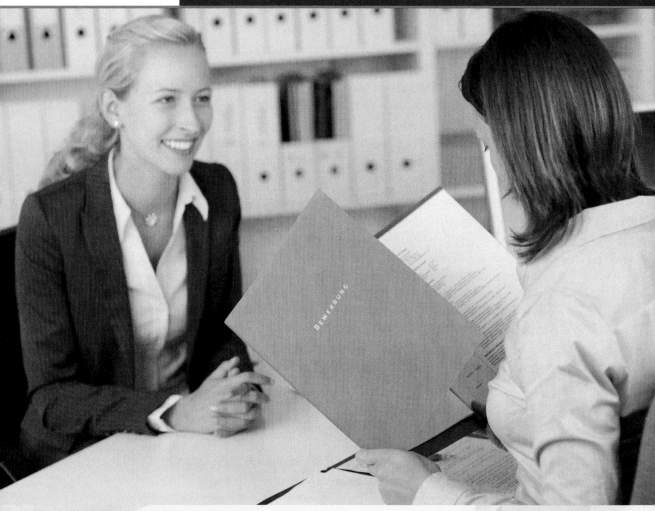

Contrastwerkstatt/Fotolia

In the practicum interview, it is important to appear professional, as well as to demonstrate confidence, interest, and a positive attitude.

INTRODUCTION

Many practicum site managers request to meet with or interview potential student-trainees before officially accepting them into the practicum arrangement in their facilities. From their perspective, this often is necessary because these professionals, while accommodating a student, still have to manage operations and account for the productivity of their facilities or departments while using time and resources to help the student meet their program's practical training objectives. Most would like to be certain in advance that the student is able to work professionally and is competent in the skills necessary to practice in the facility.

Before officially accepting a practicum arrangement, site managers and supervisors learn what they need to know about students by gathering relevant information and conducting interviews. It is during this time that they form first impressions. This chapter explores why such interviews may be required and describes numerous ways that the student can prepare for and do well in the interview. The chapter concludes with Self-Prep Questions, a Role-Play Scenario, and a Readiness Checklist.

CHAPTER OBJECTIVES

- Identify three reasons why many facility supervisors request an interview or preliminary meeting with the student candidate before accepting the training arrangement.
- Identify the possible ways a student can research (or at least become familiar with) a medical practice or health care company before his or her meeting or interview.
- List at least seven intelligent interview questions a student-trainee can ask the interviewer when prompted.
- Specify the importance of arriving at the practicum site with a professional resumé in hand.
- List at least nine rules of thumb concerning professional appearance for the interview and the practicum.
- Name three practices to be followed during the interview or preliminary meeting.
- Describe the proper method of establishing the practicum site schedule with the site manager if special scheduling is necessary.

Requests for a Preliminary Practicum Interview

You may or may not be asked to participate in an interview for your practicum. The requirement depends on the preference of the site manager who will be allowing you to practice your skills in his or her office. Some feel comfortable with any capable student walking into the office with no contact before beginning the practicum. However, many others are a bit more particular about this and feel more comfortable meeting on site for an interview before officially accepting the student for the practicum. Therefore, you should be prepared for this type of professional meeting. It is also possible that you may obtain a job directly through your practicum, and this interview may be the first step in that direction.

Reasons for a Preliminary Interview

For various specific reasons, a site manager may request an interview or some other type of introductory meeting before the practicum starts. First, an interview with the student helps the manager to assess at least three major characteristics: how well you communicate and present yourself, what professional qualities you exhibit, and how well you are likely to perform the clinical, administrative, and other practical duties specific to your specialty. These particular aspects are very important to the manager because you will be a representative of his or her organization if accepted for the practicum.

The managing staff may also request a meeting with you in order to provide you with a tour of the facility and to show you the various areas in which you will be training. Some offices already have a system to train all students that they have already established in all areas of their offices, and they may use this meeting time as an opportunity to explain their particular system of training.

This time may also be used to introduce you to other office staff who may take part in training you. As you know by now, your first in-person encounter gives the all-important first impression of you to the interviewer. Therefore, it is crucial that you consider in advance how you will present yourself with a positive attitude, confidence, and professionalism. As always, it is up to you to give your best in any meeting or interview.

Proactive Measures for Practicum Interviews

The bulk of the material presented in this chapter informs you about the ways in which you can prepare yourself for a favorable first impression in a practicum interview. The remaining sections cover the following:

- Researching the practicum site
- Submitting your resumé
- Completing application and information forms
- Presenting yourself as a professional
- Discussing your availability and setting a schedule

Researching the Site

If the medical office or facility maintains an informative Web site about the practice or the company, visit the site and commit to memory such details as the daily hours of operation, additional office locations, the number of doctors who practice on site, the medical specialties practiced in the office, and so on. This will prepare you to ask intelligent questions about the staff and the organization. It also will help you demonstrate your general interest in the patient care industry. Above all, because you have researched the organization before the interview, it will exhibit a certain level of professionalism on your part.

Typically, in interviews of any kind, you will be asked what questions, if any, you have for the interviewer. You must avoid answering "None." Always be prepared to ask at least one or two intelligent questions. Save any questions that focus on you for the end of your interview. The following questions will suffice in a medical setting:

- How long have the physicians, pharmacists, or other specialists at this office/facility been practicing?
- Do the physicians practice in this office only, or do they also see patients in a hospital or at another site?
- What procedures are performed routinely in this office?
- How many patients are seen on a daily basis by each practitioner?
- In addition to the physicians (or pharmacists, dentists, optometrists, etc.) what other patient care professionals work in this facility (e.g., physician assistants, nurse practitioners, registered nurses, medical assistants, X-ray technicians)?
- What specific credentials do you seek when hiring for a medical assisting (or other allied health) career position?
- Should you decide to accept me as a student-trainee, what are the main areas of your facility in which I will be assisting while I am completing my practicum hours?

Submitting Your Resumé

The first day you set foot in a possible or established practicum site, you should have a resumé in hand to provide to the office manager. Before that, take advantage of the resumé writing and career development resources available at your school. Your resumé is especially important because it often determines the first impression of you that the employer will develop. So, seek all the advice available to you regarding the building of a professional resumé. You will demonstrate forethought and professionalism when you have your resumé available for the site manager during the first meeting. For specific details on building an effective resumé, see Chapter 11.

Completing Application and Information Forms

The manager you meet for an interview may ask you to complete an employment application. Do not assume that this means you will be hired when you complete your practicum. Oftentimes, managers who request this of you basically prefer to see all your information in the format to which they are accustomed, knowing that it will give them the information they need. In the future, it may serve as an actual employment application, but you cannot count on this. All you can know is that the manager may or may not intend to hire you in the future and that you are expected to complete the application professionally. If this request is made of you, complete the form(s) thoroughly, accurately, and legibly.

Presenting Yourself as a Professional

Your goal in any interview, whether for the practicum or employment, is to make a positive and lasting first impression. Concerning appearances, in the medical setting it is essential to maintain personal cleanliness and professional grooming. When interviewing for the practicum as a student, you may be required to wear the uniform or scrubs and student ID that are required by your academic program or to dress in more generic interview attire. Always check with your faculty or practicum coordinator regarding the dress standards your training institution requires. The following tips apply to your practicum interview:

- Keep your scrubs (and lab coat, if required) clean and wrinkle free.
- Avoid perfume, as some patients or staff members may be sensitive to it.
- Keep makeup to a minimum. Dangling, distracting, and/or noisy jewelry should not be worn.
- If your hair is longer than shoulder length, tie it back neatly and securely.
- Keep your nails neat, clean, and short.
- Wear shoes that are clean, without holes, tears, or excessive scuffing.
- As a rule of thumb, cover any visible body piercings, jewelry, and tattoos (nose, chin, tongue, eyebrow, etc.).
- If you smoke, avoid smoking before your interview. Health care facilities are smoke free, and the status of "smoker" or "nonsmoker" may carry some weight in the decision to accept or reject you as a trainee. In other words, it is important that you do not smell of smoke while on the job. (This can also apply to employment/hiring decisions.)

These pointers may seem elementary, but you must abide by them in any professional medical or dental facility, pharmacy, or laboratory. In the event that you are asked to participate in a video or online interview, these aspects of appearance and professionalism are required at the same level as an in-person interview. Considerations for video and/or online interviewing are discussed in more detail in Chapter 11.

You also should express a desire to learn and should remember the name of the person with whom you have interviewed. Communicating in a courteous manner contributes to a professional demeanor. Any hint of an unappreciative attitude gives a first impression that is difficult to erase. Showing the medical staff that you are excited about the opportunity to learn in their office will earn you their professional respect and willingness to help you learn as much as possible. Some students forget the name of their interviewer(s), and the best and most professional way to avoid this pitfall is to obtain and briefly study the interviewer's business card during a practicum interview or on your first day as a student-trainee.

Timely arrival for your scheduled interview is also part of the first impression you give the site supervisor or interviewer. It is best to arrive approximately ten minutes before the interview. Also, if you do not know exactly

HIGHLIGHT

TIPS FROM PROFESSIONALS

Keep in mind "first impressions" when you show up to meet or interview with the site staff, manager, and provider(s). How you dress and present yourself matters; in many healthcare facilities, it is required that employees and student-trainees cover all tattoos and body piercings, aside from simple earrings. Due to our practice policies, there was an occasion when we were unable to host a student because of a tattoo.

–Office Manager (OBGYN & Primary Care group practice)

where the site is located, map it out well in advance of your appointment so that you will not arrive late. Be sure to consider traffic patterns in determining the realistic travel time you will need. Demonstrating punctuality as part of your overall first impression is a necessity.

Discussing Your Availability and Setting a Schedule

Some students need to balance the practicum with another job or unavoidable responsibility. Although such occurrences are inevitable, it is important to make yourself as available and flexible as possible for scheduling unless your school or college specifies that a full-time or other pre-established schedule must be met. Because it is important to let the site supervisor or interviewer know ahead of time whether you will need a unique set of hours for your site training, politely ask if accommodations can be made in such a circumstance. You must discuss this ahead of time so that the site staff do not expect you to conform to a schedule that you cannot possibly meet.

Many of the managers who agree to have students in the office understand the expense of being a student and that it may be necessary to keep an additional job to maintain income while in training. When attempting to schedule the maximum number of hours you think you can handle, be realistic in considering your other priorities so that you do not overestimate your availability and thus ask for a reduced schedule. Work out a schedule with the site supervisor in advance of the first day of the practicum. Once you have agreed to it, get it approved by your academic/practicum coordinator.

Keep in mind that you typically have to complete your hours within a predetermined timeframe, and thus careful planning is necessary. Your practicum syllabus and other paperwork may specify a certain number of hours weekly; if this is the case, plan according to these requirements, too. Of course, occasional times of hardship or illness leave a student no choice but to be absent from the practicum for a short time. Thus, it is important to prepare a backup plan for quickly making up any hours missed. Ask the site supervisor if, in the event of such a situation, you will be able to have an additional week on site to make up time. While dealing with everyday life, it

HIGHLIGHT

TIPS FROM PROFESSIONALS

There are a few basics to remember as you prep for an interview...appearance and first impressions are important, as well as your timeliness. Be sure your cell phone alerts are disabled during your interview time. Make sure any babysitting arrangements are secured prior to your interview day. Remember that in most medical facilities, jewelry and fragrances should be kept to minimum or avoided.

–Medical Assistant (Cardiology office)

remains very important to treat the practicum with as much priority and care as your other responsibilities, keeping in mind that it is another opportunity to make a favorable impression.

Spotlight on Pharmacy Technician Practicums

Pharmacy technician (PT) student-trainees have a rather unique role as they are often placed in a retail-store setting for the practicum. It is highly likely that the store manager and the pharmacy manager (often two different individuals) will request to meet with and interview students before offering the practicum opportunity. They will look to assess the student-applicants' professional image and abilities before allowing them to handle medications and communicate with pharmacy customers regarding medications. Beyond this, they need to determine students' ability to handle some basic business aspects of the pharmacy. PT students must demonstrate their competency up front, as pharmacies must maintain professional-grade, error-free work in filling patient prescriptions. The interviewer(s) will look for these special qualities through first impressions during the interview.

Going Above and Beyond

Before attending a practicum interview, go a step further to improve the interviewer's overall impression of you. Discuss with your instructors which certification exams you will be eligible to take upon completion of your program. Know the name of the agency that awards the certification, as well as the exact name and official abbreviation of the certification itself (e.g., CMA, RMA, NCMA, NCMOA, RHIT, CPC, RPT, NCET). Determine when you will be able to take a certification exam (see Chapter 2). When the time comes for you to discuss your professional goals with your interviewer, be prepared to describe your plans. The interviewer will then recognize your commitment to your specialty and your professional planning. (See the Appendix for the titles, abbreviations, and Web site addresses of credentialing agencies.)

Conclusion

Your overall goal for a practicum interview or any other type of pre-practicum meeting with the site manager is to make an excellent first impression so that the site staff will willingly accommodate you in their office. A positive first impression will get you off to a good start. A catchy, clear, and impressively assembled resumé will help with the first impression your interviewer forms. Be prepared with your resumé, be somewhat familiar with the facility and how it operates, and be ready to share your own professional goals confidently.

Self-Prep Questions

1. In addition to the questions cited in this chapter, what are some other intelligent questions you might ask the interviewer if you are asked to attend a practicum interview?

_____

_____

_____

_____

_____

2. Write down the resources available to you that will assist you in creating a professional resumé and in performing successfully in an interview.

_____

_____

_____

_____

_____

3. Critique yourself based on past interviews or any professional encounters, or ask a peer to take you through a mock interview. Recognize and list which aspects of interviewing are your strengths and which are your weaknesses. Think of ways to improve these weaknesses.

_____

_____

_____

_____

_____

Role-Play Scenario

Two individuals are needed for this scenario. Perform a five- to ten-minute role-play in which the interviewer asks a student-trainee candidate relevant questions about his or her experience, training, goals for the practicum, professional goals, and so on. The student-trainee being interviewed should demonstrate a working understanding of how to create a good first impression through this interview. Generally, this should include attention to appearance, mannerisms, and effective communication techniques.

1. Make a list of common interview questions (regardless of specialty), as well as a list of questions tailored to the practicum specialty (i.e., the specific field of allied health) that an interviewer can pose. Approximately five questions for each of these two areas will suffice.

_____

_____

_____

_____

_____

_____

_____

_____

_____

2. List the key areas the student-trainee candidate must consider and present during this interview process to make a positive first impression.

_____

_____

_____

_____

Readiness Checklist

_____ I am prepared for a practicum interview if I am asked to attend one.

_____ I understand why a practicum site manager probably will request an interview or preliminary meeting.

_____ I understand the benefits of researching a medical practice or company before the interview.

_____ I have committed to memory at least three intelligent questions to ask an interviewer.

_____ I have or will have my resumé prepared and updated in time for a practicum interview.

_____ I understand the basic physical appearance guidelines for the interview and the entire practicum.

_____ I understand that during the interview I am expected to be well mannered and demonstrate interest in learning more about my field.

_____ I will make it a point to remember the name of the person with whom I interview and to request a business card.

_____ I will discuss with the site manager, before the practicum, any special scheduling arrangements I will need once I am accepted for the practicum. I understand that this must also be communicated to and approved by the practicum program coordinator.

4

Attitudes and Perceptions

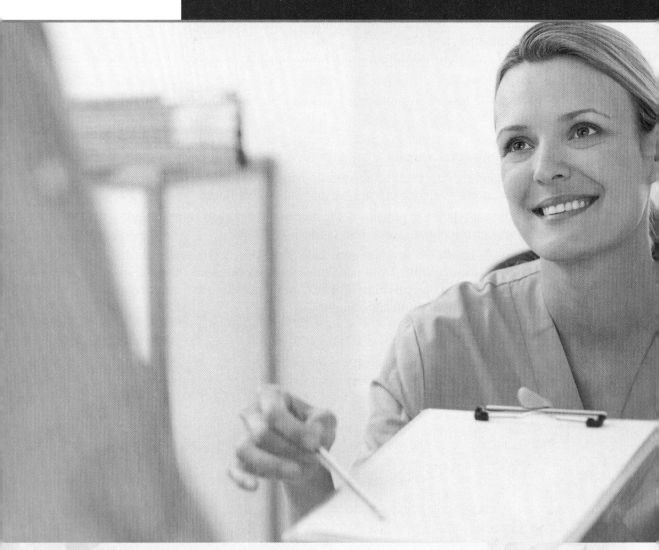

Wavebreakmedia/Shutterstock

A positive attitude is reflected by inner thoughts, outward expressions, and other aspects; overall it contributes greatly to students' ability to learn and effectively contribute while on site.

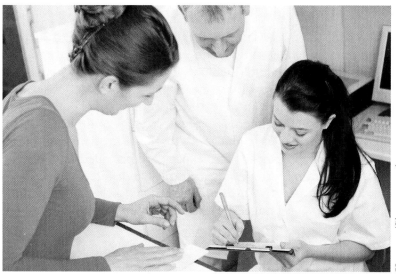

Kzenon/Shutterstock

Health care workers with positive attitudes and smiling faces contribute to patient satisfaction and cooperation.

INTRODUCTION

Perhaps the phrase "Attitude is everything" is familiar to you. People say it because attitudes profoundly influence one's success in most areas of life, especially in the professional world. Perceptions are precursors of the specific attitudes people possess. This chapter explains the connection between perceptions and attitudes and presents the most applicable recommendations and warnings as far as both are concerned. Attitudes that can ruin the practicum experience are presented with descriptions of how they can become detrimental. Positive and professionally effective attitudes can shape a productive and rewarding practicum, and these are identified with descriptions of how they can lead to success during this phase of training, as well as during your career. The chapter concludes with Self-Prep Questions, a Role-Play Scenario, and a Readiness Checklist.

CHAPTER OBJECTIVES

- List five general characteristics that contribute to an overall positive attitude.
- List five general characteristics that reflect an overall negative attitude.
- List at least five detrimental perceptions and attitudes a student might possess concerning the required practicum.
- Explain how each of the five detrimental attitudes can affect overall professional effectiveness.
- List at least four positive attitudes a student should demonstrate during the practicum.
- Explain how those four positive attitudes affect overall professional effectiveness.

Attitude and the Allied Health Practicum

Attitude is one of the most significant factors in professional success. The attitude you portray can communicate much about you, both positive and negative. This self-portrayal (defined only by you) can lead you to a fantastic start at your practicum site, or it can be the beginning of a downward spiral that may get you dismissed from your student-trainee position. A positive attitude in your training environment is characterized by optimism, friendliness, confidence, willingness to learn and gain experience in all areas of the facility, and appreciation for the training and experience provided to you. Excessive pessimism, complaining, grumpiness, self-pity, indifference, and arrogance reflect an all-around negative attitude. Contrary to the belief of some pessimists, attitudes can be changed for the better. Let's see how.

HIGHLIGHT

TIPS FROM PROFESSIONALS

The way you present yourself and come across to patients matters. Be helpful and friendly. The aura of a pleasant staff is appreciated by patients.

–Office Manager (Family Medicine Practice)

Recognizing the Human Nature of Perceptions and Attitudes

Where does an attitude come from? An experience, an expectation, someone else's influence, the media, another source? Underlying any attitude is at least one perception, which is simply your viewpoint or interpretation of an object, idea, person, or circumstance. For example, what is your attitude toward your education? How is this shaped? You might agree that it is shaped mostly by how you feel about your instructors, peers, the structure and content of the course material, and the learning environment. External factors such as how you view life and other people in general can also play a role in your attitude toward your education.

The way you see or construe your life experiences fosters the attitudes you currently hold with regard to your school or college. For example, if you feel uncomfortable with your instructors and your learning style does not connect with their teaching methods, then you likely will have an attitude of doubt and disdain. On the other hand, if your experience has been positive, with a well-equipped learning environment and instructors with whom you can relate and whose instruction you can grasp, then your attitude will likely be positive and result in personal benefit to you: You will be confident, motivated, and feel that you are progressing steadily and successfully in accomplishing your goals. Thus, it is necessary for you to be aware of how your perceptions influence your overall attitude.

Following are some of the many synonyms that show the close relation of the terms *perception* and *attitude*. Occasionally, the two are actually used as synonyms for each other; however, this analysis differentiates the two in order to observe the more outward aspect of the term *attitude* relative to the more internal aspect of *perception*:

Perception: conception, image, impression, viewpoint, insight

Attitude: character, demeanor, inclination, temperament, mental state

Attitudes are interesting because people can interpret them based on a number of features. Attitudes can be reflected by facial expressions, tone of voice, choice of words, physical mannerisms, and general behavior. Considering your upcoming entry into the health care setting, it is important to recognize that people can typically perceive attitudes in one form or another. Considering that these are determined by underlying perceptions, the starting point to change any bad attitudes for the better is through a change in perception. Some changes in this area can be challenging; others may be fairly simple. No scientific formula can be followed to change people's perceptions because each person is unique in this regard. The bottom line is that in order to change an existing negative perception, one must first recognize the need for the change and be motivated to change it. This works most of the time when people realize that it would be beneficial for them to adopt a more positive approach to life situations while letting go of the negative perceptions that cripple their chances of success. As a student-trainee, it is to your benefit personally and professionally to examine your attitudes and trace those needing improvement to the perceptions that shape them.

This chapter first discusses what specific perceptions and attitudes are detrimental, followed by a discussion of the kind of approach that will lead to success at your site. As you read, keep in mind that the attitude you portray can positively or negatively influence your success in working with medical professionals and patients.

Changing Detrimental Attitudes and Perceptions

To get the most out of your practicum, it is important to have the right attitude. Thus, certain perceptions will be detrimental to you and your experience and, therefore, should be avoided. The following are examples of such perceptions.

Detrimental Perception #1: "I provide free labor."

You must not believe during the practicum that you provide free labor for someone's business. Convincing yourself of this false notion will damage your overall attitude. For one thing, an "unpaid" practicum is mandated by many allied health accrediting and credentialing agencies, such as the American Association of Medical Assistants (AAMA). Also, during your practicum, you are not doing the site staff a favor; rather, the site staff are doing you a favor. During this phase, you are not considered to be an independent, qualified professional because you do not yet possess an adequate level of experience. You have not yet graduated officially from your program, and chances are that you have not yet had the opportunity to sit for a credentialing exam.

The practicum is an integral part of your training, and you are the one with the most to gain from it. In addition, because of the initial training that must be provided, a practicum student's presence often reduces the staff's productivity for a time. You should view your practicum as the site staff's sacrifice for your benefit, and you should express an attitude of gratitude. Your trainers and supervisors will quickly sense whether your attitude is positive or negative.

The following constitutes the components of this detrimental perception:

- *The detrimental perception:* "I am free labor. This manager only wants to use me for free work. Why should I work for free?"
- *Signs of the detrimental attitude:* Outward signs of dismay, such as a disgruntled demeanor and lack of motivation.
- *The realization:* "This supervisor or staff member is taking time out to help me learn and be successful. It is good and charitable of managers and employees to help budding allied health professionals gain appropriately guided experience."
- *The good perception:* "I see the value in what I am being offered through the practicum and will appreciate it and take with me new experiences necessary for my professional growth."
- *Signs of a good attitude:* Willingness to learn, satisfaction in the practicum experience, resulting in a happy vibe, expressions of thankfulness, and good customer service.

Detrimental Perception #2: "I performed well in school, so I am an expert."

The belief that you have already mastered and become an expert in your respective allied health specialty just because you performed well in school is another perception that will not earn you one iota of respect. You have many practical lessons (both technical and professional) to learn outside of the classroom setting. This is not to be confused with possessing confidence in your work; display confidence by all means but not a know-it-all or haughty attitude. Yes, you deserve much credit for your classroom attendance and hard-earned grades, but this is far from the completion of your education.

You should pursue the practicum for what it truly is: another new course in your curriculum. Look carefully at your school's course description for the practicum. Also read the syllabus for the course objectives and the description of what is expected of you, as you would for any course. Only after you successfully complete the practicum should you pat yourself on the back for completing the full spectrum of your training.

Furthermore, you may choose to obtain an even higher qualification— that is, one or more of several credentialing and certification exams—that will prove your expertise. Even beyond this, nothing on paper (certificates, diplomas, degrees, or professional memberships) compares to the expertise of an experienced professional. Once you achieve that level, which takes much time and hard work, then you will have good reason to consider yourself a fully qualified professional or expert in your field. When you eventually become a credentialed and experienced professional, be sure that your success does not prompt you to form an attitude of arrogance as this will surely diminish your professional reputation.

The following constitute the components of this detrimental perception:

- *The detrimental perception:* "I already know everything I need to know. There is not much the practicum experience can offer me."
- *Signs of the detrimental attitude:* The haughty, know-it-all attitude, which others see as arrogance; inability to take constructive criticism; difficulty in functioning as a team player; irritation when others try to help you.
- *The realization:* "The practicum is a new experience, where my skills will be tested and refined in a real-world setting with the help and guidance of health care professionals. It will be completely different from the classroom experience and a beneficial challenge."
- *The good perception:* "I will be actively learning and practicing in the presence of genuine professionals. They will help me to cultivate the professionalism expected in this field and to further refine my skills. This is all to my benefit."
- *Signs of a good attitude:* Confidence in existing skills, readiness to ask for advice to improve your skills, and finding value in what your peers and supervisor(s) contribute to your learning.

Detrimental Perception #3: "Practicum? Whatever. . . . "

A laissez-faire attitude is unacceptable. If you demonstrate a blasé mind-set, those supervising you will know that you are not interested in what you are doing and that you will not be a valuable asset to their team, or to any other medical team or office to which they might otherwise refer you for future employment. If you are the type of student who is overly relaxed or indifferent, with no sense of urgency when it comes to getting tasks done in a timely manner, and getting them done right, then you should ponder this aspect of yourself and devise a plan for improvement. Medical offices and other facilities are typically in hustle mode each and every day as they tend to patients and customers. There is no need for an extra person who has no business but to linger around unproductively during a busy schedule. Students can be and have been dismissed permanently from sites for showing this nonchalant and disinterested attitude. (Remember that such dismissal from a site will impact your grade.)

Indifference is also an attitude that can be easily detected in any type of interview or first meeting, so consider this ahead of time. It may be comfortable for you to take your time doing things, with no sense of urgency, and there may be nothing wrong with this as a personality trait and in your leisure time. However, in patient care and customer-focused facilities, this cannot be the attitude you present, whether as a student-trainee or an employee. Productivity is expected no matter what area of allied health you are pursuing.

The following constitute the components of this detrimental perception:

- *The detrimental perception:* "This is boring. Oh well, whatever, there's no hurry. I'll just wait until somebody gives me instructions. It does not really matter what I do anyway, as long as I am at the site."
- *Signs of the detrimental attitude:* Disinterest in your career field, lack of initiative or drive to work, appearing lazy or bored or both.
- *The realization:* "There is no tolerance for laziness or lack of productivity in a patient care setting. Nobody will consider employing a person demonstrating these characteristics, not to mention consideration for career promotion."
- *The good perception:* "There is a standard of care and professionalism that must be maintained, and I will rise to the challenge of the rapid pace and diligence involved in all areas of health care."
- *Signs of a good attitude:* Readiness to work, efficient and effective work habits, asking questions and seeking advice, taking initiative in all possible situations, and offering help to others.

Detrimental Perception #4: "My personal problems are more than I can manage today."

Arriving to work with an obviously grumpy or unhappy attitude because of personal problems will be noticed, and you then run the risk of being perceived unfavorably. Leave behind all your personal problems once you are at the training site. For some people, this intention must be given thought well in advance. Most of us have various types of personal problems and pressures to deal with constantly: children, relationships, finances, and so on. Many people you will work with also have their share of issues, but they keep their jobs by showing up with the intention to do one thing: their job.

If your personal life is not going well, make a complete success out of your practicum! If all else is failing, make this your time to shine and improve professionally; deal with your personal problems at another time. Do not let your issues get in the way of reporting to your site daily and on time. You should acquire this habit before you enter the workforce; practicing it seriously during the practicum is imperative.

The following constitute the components of this detrimental perception:

- *The detrimental perception:* "I have so many problems to deal with, and I am so stressed. Spending a whole day at the practicum just adds to it all. I cannot cope."
- *Signs of the detrimental attitude:* Distraction from working and learning, not acting professionally because of lack of focus and concentration.
- *The realization:* "The practicum is short term, and it will benefit my professional growth to suppress the stress of other life issues while at the site so that I can learn and succeed and demonstrate to others that I am fully capable of professional-level work."
- *The good perception:* "This is easy enough. I simply need to shift my focus during on-site training hours. I can and will present myself pleasantly and professionally. I can deal with my problems later."
- *Signs of a good attitude:* Ability to focus on work, a calm and pleasant demeanor, and others (patients and staff) feel confident and comfortable with your work.

Detrimental Perception #5: "Something's always wrong."

If you tend to complain, now is the time to recognize that complaining is taboo in any professional office or facility. You can rid yourself of this tendency by setting the intention to improve this attitude.

If you complain often, chances are that you probably are not seeing enough of the good in life. Think about how it appears to staff members and patients when you complain. The staff at your practicum site may assume that you do not appreciate the accommodation being made for you, and you may lose your position. Patients may feel uncomfortable if they hear complaining because they seek care coupled with competence and professionalism—a worker's complaining undermines both of these.

If by nature you are a pessimist, intentionally shifting your focus to the positive aspects of life will require substantial effort on your part. It is to your benefit that your desire to succeed in your new career is likely to provide sufficient motivation for you to seriously put effort into this change. In fact, keeping your eye on the goal of succeeding in your career should be the underlying motivator for following all the advice provided in this guide, as well as other sources intended to assist you.

The following constitute the components of this detrimental perception:

- *The detrimental perception:* "Why do bad things always happen to me? Nothing ever turns out right or good for me."
- *Signs of the detrimental attitude:* Frequent dissatisfaction, overreaction to minor inconveniences, recognizing and pointing out the faults of others, general appearance of unhappiness, customer service ability suffers.

- *The realization:* "Complaining will not help me in my professional endeavors. I can change this aspect of myself."
- *The good perception:* "Resolving not to complain, especially in a professional environment, raises my level of professionalism and effectiveness."
- *Signs of a good attitude:* Ease and a positive attitude in adapting to inconvenient situations, quick to seek solutions rather than complaining about the problem.

Attitudes that Promote Productivity and Success

By approaching your practicum with the right attitude, you not only will be more helpful at your site but also will reap more benefits from the experience. Ways you can achieve this include the following:

- Caring for others
- Committing to serve
- Using good manners
- Showing enthusiasm

Caring for Others

Having chosen a division of allied health for your career, possessing a genuinely caring attitude toward people should be quite natural for you and your peers. You have chosen to be part of a team that is dedicated to caring for and serving patients and customers—hence, the frequently heard terms *patient care* and *customer service*, aiming toward the goal of *patient and customer satisfaction.* This attitude should be present in all your professional encounters with staff and patients.

A patient or customer will become uncomfortable as soon as he or she does not feel that sense of caring coming from you (or any other staff member). Patients with problems are very sensitive to how they are treated in the medical establishment. They are even sensitive to this treatment in other situations, such as when discussing their issues over the phone with office staff, when visiting an outside facility for lab work, and when interacting with pharmacy staff about medications or insurance coverage. So put on a warm smile and use a gentle, concerned voice at all times, even when you may not be in the best mood. You will benefit, too, by feeling the effects of positively impacting somebody else's day.

Committing to Serve

Make it your duty to serve, knowing that serving others with a positive and caring attitude is far reaching, for both you and those you serve. Leaders do not become leaders until they first serve others. Is your goal to advance into positions such as department head, office manager, or clinical manager? Or are you looking to be paid on the high end of the pay scale when you have more experience? If so, your service to others will guide you there in due time. Even when you achieve your goal of becoming a clinic, department, or office manager, or holding some other advanced position, you will be serving others even more, not just receiving more pay, prestige, and recognition.

The quality of service you provide to others (patients or staff) is determined significantly by your attitude. If your attitude is that everyone should cater to you (or serve your needs) and that you are supposed to be the center of attention, then your service to others will be minimal or nonexistent. If your attitude is that you chose your particular profession because you want to help others and you truly see the great value in doing so, then you will be among those who provide the most effective and recognized service. Others in your working environment will quickly and easily grasp and remember this about you. Therefore, it is in your best interest to make the conscious decision— before you begin your practicum—to show this attitude of friendly service.

Using Good Manners

It is very important that you *use good manners*. This seems elementary— perhaps it is something you learned in childhood and still value. However, a handful of adults and even highly educated people in the working world have not mastered the general rules of polite social conduct. Perhaps they work in professions where these skills are unnecessary, but in patient care and customer service the use of good manners is essential to demonstrate concern and respect for others. Good manners are the foundation of excellent customer service, and they reassure patients that they are well cared for and respected by those providing their health services.

The patients with whom you interact will expect politeness and respect from you, and your superiors in the office will respect you more when they see you demonstrating this to them and others. The same applies when communicating by telephone, whether you are setting appointments, calling in prescriptions or lab work, scheduling a surgery, speaking with a patient or customer, or resolving issues with an insurance agent. Thus, saying "Please," "Thank you," "Excuse me," and so on is necessary at all times. If your normal, daily vocabulary does not already include these pleasantries, practice and train yourself to use them regularly. Your mannerisms and demeanor represent you, as well as the entire office or facility in which you are working and your school.

Showing Enthusiasm

Enthusiasm is a positive attitude that will help you in achieving your goals. Are you enthusiastic about starting your career? Are you motivated to learn and accrue experience? Are you excited that you will have many opportunities to help people in need? And will those working with you and those you are serving be able to see this aspect of you in your day-to-day performance? Not only can you brighten the day of others through your enthusiasm for your work, but you also thereby help yourself to be perceived by others as a trainee, and eventually a professional, who is content and confident.

Enthusiasm can boost the overall quality of your work. Patient and customer satisfaction remain priorities throughout all areas of health care, and enthusiastic workers who help achieve this goal are sought after by all employers.

HIGHLIGHT

TIPS FROM PROFESSIONALS

In our practice, we strongly believe in the power of a positive attitude...the right attitude contributes greatly to your progress and achievements, it also impacts others in beneficial ways. We make sure this carries over to our patients from the start, as well as through every visit and point of follow up we have with them. An attitude of service is a necessity for anyone working in healthcare, especially students in training.

–Office Coordinator (Pediatrics office)

Developing Perceptions and Attitudes at the Practicum Site

You should seriously consider the preceding discussion of perceptions and attitudes before the practicum begins. This section touches upon those perceptions that you might possibly develop once you have begun to take notice of the behaviors of other staff members during your practicum. It is not intended to generalize and make assumptions about staff ahead of time but, rather, to raise general awareness.

The following scenarios are simply examples. These types of concerns do not present themselves in all practicum experiences. You may find that they assist you as you consider perceptions and attitudes at your training site.

1. You are in a different position than those working around you at the site. You are the student or the apprentice, not an employee who has been with the organization for a while. If an employee is demonstrating practices that are unprofessional or commonly discouraged while at work (talking on a cell phone, searching the Internet, paying personal bills, gossiping, and so on), take it upon yourself to have the sense *not* to

exhibit that behavior. Just because you perceive that you are in a relaxed or nonchalant environment, as a student-trainee you cannot assume any attitude or action that you observe, such as minimizing your effort because others do so. You must always draw professional boundaries for yourself and abide by them.

2. You may perceive that employees around you are talking about you behind your back. Although this is possible, do not retaliate with any type of negative attitude or action. If you can ignore it and concentrate only on your work, do so. If it bothers you and interferes with your ability to work or concentrate, seek advice from the manager or supervisor and, if appropriate, your school's practicum coordinator or liaison. In this scenario, it is important to avoid wrongly accusing others simply because you have "a feeling" that they have acted in this way. Remember your position at the site as a student-trainee: Do not exhibit any negative attitude or reaction that will put you in a bad position.

3. You notice after your first week or two that the general tendency among some people you are working with is to be caught up in office politics. When you observe this type of drama, do not become involved, even if you feel that anyone is attempting to get you involved. If given any opportunity to respond to this—don't. If you are asked for your opinion or to get involved in any way in such situations, simply and politely reply that you wish not to be involved because of your student status. Remember: Your professionalism counts toward your final practicum grade.

Give your attention immediately to any negative perceptions you realize you are developing. You do not want to develop an attitude that might cause you further problems. If you cannot check any negative perceptions you are developing on your own, speak with your school practicum coordinator or liaison about the issue. Many times, simply discussing the scenario and listening to another's insight will help clear your vision and restore appropriate perceptions.

Spotlight on Medical Administrative Assistant/ Medical Office Specialist Practicums

As the first point of contact for arriving patients or customers, or for callers making contact with the medical office by phone, the medical administrative assistant or medical office specialist student-trainee—in order to create a good first impression—must portray a positive attitude. This individual must come across as truly desiring to assist each incoming patient, showing a level of care and concern that makes patients feel welcomed and important. Smiling often and speaking in a pleasant tone contribute to the outward expression of a positive attitude on the job.

Conclusion

The attitude and perception considerations presented in this chapter are major contributors to successful practicum experiences. To maintain a positive attitude, focus on the positive aspects of life and, especially, on your commitment to succeeding in your career. Be a critic of your own strengths and weaknesses, and adjust your outlook accordingly. Your attitudes and perceptions greatly influence how you work and how professional you are. During your practicum, be positive, appreciative, respectful, and willing to learn from your mentors.

Self-Prep Questions

1. Evaluate yourself. What attitude traits do you possess that will afford you a positive practicum experience? What are some areas you think you should improve on before your practicum?

   _____

   _____

   _____

   _____

   _____

2. If you were interviewing a student-trainee to work with your medical office team, what attitudes would you seek in that person?

   _____

   _____

   _____

   _____

   _____

3. In previous positions or jobs you have held, what attitudes do you recall that made your peers, co-workers, or managers respectable and recognized workers?

   _____

   _____

   _____

   _____

   _____

Role-Play Scenario

This scenario requires three individuals:

- *The student-trainee,* who can be any type of allied health worker; simply adjust the role and content as needed
- *The customer or patient* who encounters this student
- *The site supervisor* who oversees the student and is the point of contact for the school's practicum coordinator

The three individuals perform two short scenarios to reflect opposing ends of the attitude spectrum. The student-trainee will decide whether to first act out the positive or the negative attitude. The direction the scenario takes will be based on how the student-trainee acts.

Open the scene with initial contact being made between the customer or patient and the student. For example, if the student is a medical assistant (MA), the scene could start with the MA calling the patient from the waiting area to the patient room. As another example, if the student is a front office, billing, or pharmacy tech trainee, the patient or customer could walk up to the desk to discuss a question or issue. More specifically, for a pharmacy scenario the pharmacy technician trainee may assist a patient at the desk who has a question about a medication or about their insurance benefits covering a certain medication. In a medical front office scenario, the administrative specialist may assist a patient with questions regarding insurance benefits, rescheduling an appointment, payments, or account balance.

In two separate scenes, the student should portray traits to create the negative attitude and the positive attitude. Participants should try not to overact and simply to play out what realistic attitudes can show, both positive and negative.

The third individual (the student's supervisor) sees and hears the encounter between the customer or patient and the student and then speaks to the student-trainee concerning the attitude he or she portrayed in the encounter. These could be words of encouragement or reprimand, depending on which attitude scenario took place.

1. What are some realistic positive and negative attitudes that can be portrayed by the student? Give at least three examples of each.

_____

_____

_____

_____

_____

2. In each of the opposing scenarios, how would the student's attitudes affect his or her ability to perform basic job duties well and to serve the patient or customer effectively?

_____

_____

_____

_____

_____

3. In each of the opposing scenarios, how would the student's attitude affect the patient or customer?

_____

_____

_____

_____

_____

4. In each of the opposing scenarios, what are the various ways the student-trainee could expect the supervisor to handle the attitudes portrayed?

_____

_____

_____

_____

_____

5. How can these attitudes affect the success and grade for the student's practicum?

_____

_____

_____

_____

_____

6. How can the opposing attitudes affect the chances of the student becoming employed through the practicum or being referred for employment to another facility?

_____

_____

_____

_____

_____

Readiness Checklist

_____ I recognize how my perceptions in certain areas directly influence my attitudes.

_____ I understand the likely pitfalls of possessing detrimental attitudes during my practicum.

_____ I understand how the right attitudes can influence my overall success.

_____ I have identified any personal perceptions I possess that may become problematic.

_____ I have considered ways to overcome problematic perceptions for my practicum term.

_____ I understand how my attitudes can affect the patients or customers I will serve.

_____ I know that I have the willpower to leave behind any personal issues or problems while at my practicum site.

_____ I understand that I am still a student and am subject to the procedures and techniques recommended or required at my site.

_____ I can follow all required procedures and techniques with a positive attitude.

_____ I recognize the necessity of using good manners in the patient care and customer service settings.

5

Etiquette and Professional Manners

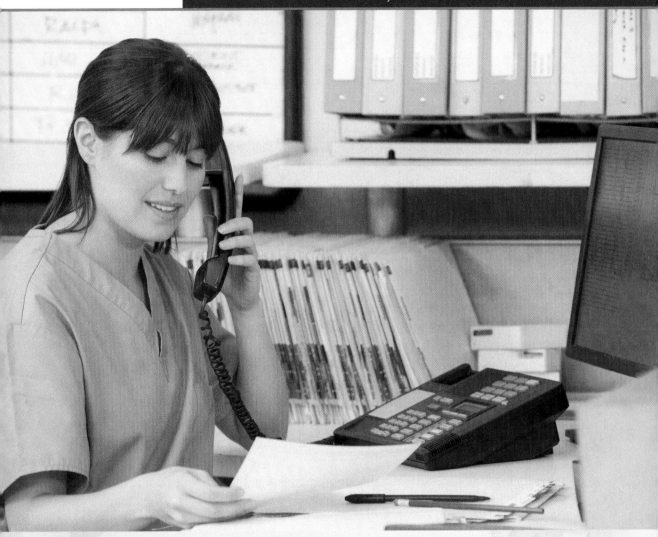

Shutterstock

It is important to practice professional etiquette when assisting patients in person and on the phone, as well as when working as part of a team.

INTRODUCTION

This chapter highlights the importance of using professional manners and avoiding unprofessional ones. Manners, and the lack thereof, say much about a person and can communicate both favorable and unfavorable characteristics. Several aspects of etiquette are well worth the attention of all allied health students entering the health care industry. Once identified, each point of etiquette is described in light of how it communicates various messages at the practicum site. This discussion also demonstrates how correcting these tendencies can contribute to professional development while you avoid behavior-related pitfalls during the practicum. The chapter concludes with Self-Prep Questions, a Role-Play Scenario, and a Readiness Checklist.

CHAPTER OBJECTIVES

- Identify the general meaning of the term *etiquette*.
- Identify the importance of appropriate etiquette in the allied health practicum.
- Identify at least three aspects that your posture can communicate.
- Name at least six additional manners that affect how others view you professionally.
- Explain the appropriate way(s) to deal with each of those six additional manners.
- Name at least four distracting behaviors that affect your professional demeanor.
- Explain at least one possible solution for each of those four distracting behaviors.
- Identify five ways to retain a "clean" image within social media.

The Significance of Etiquette

Etiquette generally refers to the various manners and behaviors prescribed by and observed in social life. How do you carry yourself? How do you portray your work ethic? How can others see that you are committed to your work and concerned about the welfare of patients and customers? These traits are all categorized within the context of your personal etiquette. It speaks to others about you in many ways: how you work, whether you genuinely care, whether you are a committed worker, and so on. You can show utmost respect for others and professionalism through your personal set of manners, and it is crucial to recognize which manners, habits, and gestures are not acceptable in any professional setting, even while you are a student. Every person has his or her own unique set of manners that includes positive and negative (or unfavorable or unprofessional) aspects. Sometimes socially unacceptable behavior is perceived as acceptable. Many people, even those who are highly educated or have a long history of successful work experience, may benefit from tweaking their manners a bit to optimize their professional demeanor.

Students have been permanently dismissed from their training sites for behaving in an unacceptable manner, as well as for their attitude issues. Thus, this entire chapter is devoted to the single topic of etiquette. Both acceptable and unacceptable manners are discussed. Self-presentation through posture, verbal manners, and professional language is analyzed, and basic tips on behavior are included.

Several particular aspects of your character say much about you, your confidence, abilities, and interests. For example, I worked with a student who was dismissed from two different sites for the same reasons. She had no problems arriving on time or doing as she was instructed, but her unprofessional demeanor and etiquette were more than what the managers at the two practicum sites were willing to tolerate. In this case, the main issues were not smiling (appearing grumpy), waiting to be told what to do (not taking initiative), slouching when sitting, leaning when standing, chewing gum, and showing an overall disinterest in learning. This combination communicated that this student was not motivated, did not care about the staff or patients, and did not appear to have the potential to be a productive worker. The site managers indicated that this style simply does not work in a health care setting.

In summary, even if your skills and techniques are superb in the classroom, personal aspects matter during the practicum just as much as your technical competencies. In addition, it is important to pay attention to etiquette as you prepare for job interviews—it determines much of the interviewer's first impression of you.

Etiquette for Allied Health Student-Trainees and Professionals

Several aspects of etiquette that will be important to focus on during your practicum include the following:

- Posture
- Verbal manners
- Word choice
- Avoiding distracting behaviors

Posture

Your posture says much about you. It reflects your confidence level and your attitude, as well as your interest in what is happening around you. If you slouch in chairs or lean frequently on desks and countertops, do you think the people around you will perceive you as a confident and effective or productive worker? Actually, they will wonder what is wrong with you and may even think you are experiencing physical discomfort or pain. Patients will think like that, too, and this will have important implications. Patients need to feel that they are being cared for by a high-quality and confident health care team, not by people who drag themselves around and twiddle their thumbs or who appear not to know what is going on. Patients and others who have business at the practicum site are more comfortable and satisfied with staff members who show interest, demonstrate care, and carry themselves professionally.

A poor or negative attitude can often lead a person to slouch, and the look of slouching or dragging oneself about tends to repel people, especially if this posture is a chronic habit. Typically, this posture also reflects boredom, unproductiveness, and even lack of a work ethic.

There is a general correlation between attitude and posture (of course, with the exception of any medical condition affecting the spine/vertebrae). Thus, changing one's posture comes more easily to those who make a conscious effort to change the underlying perceptions and attitudes that originally led to persistently slouching and leaning. (To review the importance of attitudes and perceptions, see Chapter 4.)

Disinterest in performing everyday duties and learning as you work can easily convince others, including facility managers and physicians, that you may not be truly committed to your chosen career field. As a student-trainee, demonstrating a lack of interest in your practicum will not serve you well when it comes to your evaluation by the site manager or the opportunity to initiate professional contacts and relationships to jump-start your career. It is very important to assess your behavior to ensure that you actually are communicating what you want to about yourself during the practicum.

Verbal Manners

The level of professionalism you display with your verbal manners and associated tactics also affects how others view you professionally. These manners and tactics include how you speak to others, your listening skills, ability to apologize, manner of addressing conflicts, and generally how you treat others. Consider the following specifics:

- Using manners as a mechanism of showing a favorable attitude was discussed in Chapter 4. The use of good manners should become natural for professional people hoping to be successful. It shows consideration and respect for other staff members, customers, and patients.
- Speaking like a professional practitioner is another direct indicator of how professional you are in your field. This skill involves understanding and applying vocabulary pertaining to your specialty and avoiding the use of unprofessional fillers, such as *uh*, *um*, and *like*, while communicating. (See the next section for examples of casual and improper phrases and their professional translations.) Keep a medical terminology book or medical dictionary handy so that you can easily check your use of professional medical terms. Your work team and patients form a more respectful perception of you and are confident in you when you speak professionally.

- During the communication process, it is of utmost importance to steer clear of any tendency to interrupt when someone else is speaking. This tendency is sometimes irresistible, such as when you are convinced that the message being communicated merits correcting.
- Correcting or adding to somebody else's words or comments must be done tactfully. Never correct a team member or engage in a confrontation in the presence of a patient or customer.
- It is a known fact that not a single person is perfect, and therefore, if you happen to make a mistake or handle something incorrectly, admit your fault and apologize. Also, state your intention of not making the same mistake again and, if possible, thank the person who pointed out your error. We tend to despise people who constantly correct us, but these corrections and what we learn from them build us professionally.
- When addressing conflicts, the best approach is to address them as situation related rather than person related. In other words, focus on the problem's aspects and seeking a solution rather than on anyone's faults and communicating your opinions to others. Engaging in the latter is a sign of immaturity and lack of professionalism. Also, addressing conflict from the situation-related viewpoint helps in reducing or eliminating further interpersonal issues related to the issue at hand.
- A reliable and relevant rule of thumb, often referred to as the golden rule, is to treat others the way you wish to be treated. This means extending courteousness, forgiveness, encouragement, empowerment, compliments, recognition, and the like to others at the appropriate times. Aren't these what you hope others will extend to you?

Word Choice

It is important to employ grammatically proper, professional, and polite language in any professional setting, especially in allied health professions. Would you like to be acknowledged and respected as a professional? If so, your wording and tone of voice are as important as the array of other factors noted. Table 5-1 ■ provides a short list of selected example phrases, along with the appropriate way to say the same thing in a professional environment. You will see that a few of these focus on the matter of tone, whereas others address proper use of the English language. As other phrases come to mind, perhaps you will recognize them and be able to think quickly of the more professionally acceptable wording and tone.

Avoiding Distracting Behaviors

Some distracting behaviors and conditions should be avoided while in the professional environment. The following points delineate a few of them that are important, along with some recommendations.

Table 5.1 ■ Word Choice

Unprofessional Wording and Phrase	The Professional Alternative
What? Huh?	Pardon? Excuse me?
Yah.	Yes.
Nah.	No.
What's up?	How are you?
What do you need?	How may I help you?
You ain't got . . . ?	Do you not have . . . ?
I ain't . . .	I do not . . .
I don't understand anything you just said.	Please clarify what you mean.
We don't got none.	We don't have any.

- In a medical facility, pharmacy, hospital, or billing office, and especially during the practicum, you should never chew gum. In fact, the office or facility rules for staff likely include a written policy against it. It is offensive to some staff, customers, and patients, and the act of chewing gum does not fit the image of a clean and sanitary medical or professional environment.

   It is important not to have bad breath when working in close contact with others, but this can be achieved though proper dental care and not by chewing gum. A thorough brush, floss, and rinse are appropriate before work. Breath mints after snacks and lunch also are useful. Some foods, particularly sulfurous foods such as garlic, cabbage, and onions, should always be avoided before working around others, as these cause bad breath.

- At times other than during a formal break, snack items should be consumed where designated and out of the sight of patients or customers. Food, wrappers, snack bags, soda cans, and the like diminish the image of a neat and sanitary medical environment. On occasions when a snack or tray of food is provided in the break area, you should demonstrate appropriate etiquette by taking a reasonable or small amount, even if you are very hungry. Be considerate of others who may come along after you for their portions. The best behavior is to wait until the regular employees have had their chance to take what they would like before you. This is simply the courteous and respectful way to act in this situation. In addition, be sure to clean up after consuming food or drink on site.

- Another very important point to consider is that a practitioner who works in very close proximity to patients and customers should never smell of cigarette smoke while on duty; this is highly offensive to some staff members and patients. This particular odor also works against the goal of a clean and sanitary working environment.

- Do not appear tired. If excessive fatigue is an issue on any given day, it is important to find ways to cope rather than showing such obvious signs as constantly yawning or resting your head in any way. Be sure you allow yourself enough nighttime sleep, as you will likely work full days during the practicum. While at your site, if necessary, ask to take a brief break, go outside, and take a three- to five-minute walk in partial sunlight to re-energize. Consuming fruit and other types of healthy snacks, especially with substantial protein content, during the day (rather than snacks like chips and cookies) also helps to maintain your energy level.

- All phones and other portable devices, such as tablets, should be turned off or silenced while at the practicum site. These devices should not be visible to other staff or to patients and customers. Trying to squeeze in personal time on one's devices while on the job is viewed as unprofessional, and if perceived as a habit by the site supervisor, it may be another potential reason for permanent dismissal from the site. It is usually acceptable to use these devices when officially off the clock or on break time. If use of these devices is allowed during break times in designated areas, be sure that you remain professional in your activity while anywhere on the site's property. In other words, it is best to avoid streaming videos, playing music, or visiting questionable or inappropriate Web sites. Make sure you fully understand the rules at your site concerning this issue. In any case, one definite rule of thumb is to not use these devices anywhere patients or customers can see you.

- Regarding computer use at the practicum site, just because you have been placed at a computer station to complete certain tasks does not mean that it is okay to use the Internet for any personal reasons or to play computer games. This includes checking personal e-mail, paying bills, shopping, checking social media, and so on. Computer games can be habitual for some people when no immediate task is at hand. These games must be avoided as well, especially when, as a student-trainee, you are attempting to make your best impression on the professionals training you.

During the practicum, it is imperative to give your best effort in all areas. Consider what personal adjustments are necessary, and plan ahead to be successful. The preceding recommendations cover some of the most common areas of concern for students to consider before the practicum.

Spotlight on the Surgical Technology Practicum

Surgery patients rely on the comfort and reassurance they receive from their surgical team. At a time when these patients can be somewhat apprehensive, such as on their way into the operating room, the competence and caring nature of the surgeon(s) and their team of surgical technologists and nurses must resonate with the patient. Professional etiquette throughout the pre-op procedures, along with the surgical team's effective bedside manner, can make a difference in how comfortable and calm the patient feels and how he or she will perceive the care received, even in the post-op phase. Important aspects that stand out to surgery patients are the demeanor of the surgical team as well as the way the team members communicate with the patient and with each other. The surgery experience for the patient becomes more positive when they see these qualities during such an uncertain and possibly emotional time.

Social Media Etiquette and Behavior

Believe it or not, the social media channels (Facebook, Twitter, Snapchat, Instagram, etc.) can be and are used by employers to provide a glimpse into the personal nature of potential student-trainees and employees, and even current employees, especially those being considered for promotions. Certain employers are concerned about the overall personality and nature of individuals involved with their organizations in addition to their professional qualifications and experience. Checking into social media sites provides insight when the character of a person is important for the position or promotion in question. Therefore, as aspiring health care professionals, it is up to all practicum (and job) candidates to consider their personal presentation in social media.

Social media use includes communication through both language and visual images, so it is necessary to create a positive image of oneself through what is said in writing and posted in the form of photos or videos on one's page/site/timeline. The idea is not necessarily to speak and act professionally within these platforms but, rather, simply to avoid any content that would create doubt or raise questions as to the appropriateness of how personal time is spent.

The following are some tips for keeping a "clean" image within social media:

- Avoid images that are inappropriate. Profile images, for example, should be a photo you are comfortable showing to a family member or boss/manager at your job.
- Avoid slang as much as possible. Communicating too much in this type of lingo creates the impression that your written communication skills may not be on par with professional correspondence and documentation.
- Avoid bad language, such as profanities and terms that reflect hatred or anger. When this type of language is associated with you, it conveys personal instability and lack of self-control.
- Avoid negativity in your attitude toward life. This shows through your written content. Sometimes it is okay to be honest if you are posting

to friends that you had a bad day, but showing the down side of life regularly or often can make it appear that you lack a positive outlook and tend to stay stuck in problems, which may affect your ability to focus and be productive.

• Avoid any inappropriate written content. In determining what qualifies as inappropriate, simply consider whether you would want your family members or potential employers to come across the content you post. If it is not something you would share with them, then it is best to keep it off the site.

Keeping your social media activities free of questionable content will help employers develop a good impression of your personal life when it matters or is important to a certain position or to an organization's overall vision and mission in serving patients and/or customers.

HIGHLIGHT

TIPS FROM PROFESSIONALS

Always present yourself as professional - this includes how you speak as well as how you appear. Show up on time to the site each day looking neat and clean. You are pursuing your career, so make sure you reflect a professional image in all aspects.

–Medical Assistant (Cardiology office)

Conclusion

These aspects of etiquette are significant as you enter the allied health industry. The more personal contact and communication you have with patients, customers, and other health care professionals, the more important your manners become. The best way to ensure a good start is to visualize yourself working with patients or customers in the setting and to zoom in to the impressions being developed about you as their service or care provider. Think carefully about what areas you may need to improve upon before beginning your practicum so that you do not have any etiquette issues interfering with your professional performance.

Self-Prep Questions

1. Name at least five behaviors or manners that are unacceptable.

_____

_____

_____

_____

_____

2. What aspects of etiquette do you feel you should improve on for your practicum?

_____

_____

_____

_____

_____

3. What are your etiquette strengths? How do you think these will promote you as a professional in your allied health specialty?

_____

_____

_____

_____

_____

4. What social media site(s) do you use? How do you feel about the content they contain? Do you think that you need to change any aspects of your online etiquette so that your personal life appears more appealing to potential employers or site managers who check in for further insight?

_____

_____

_____

_____

_____

Role-Play Scenario

This scenario requires four to ten individuals, depending on class size (more if feasible). An audience is also needed to actively critique the created scene. The scenario is an office party for a physician's birthday. The office is usually closed daily for the lunch hour, which is when the party is being held in the facility's break room. Set up a table with snacks and beverages for the celebration. One to three students can be designated as the student-trainees, while the others participating in the scenario are the employees. The group performing should act out the office party scene, focusing on proper etiquette but at the same time carrying on with normal eating, conversation, and interaction with others. The audience should have paper and pen readily available during the scene to critique observable etiquette and to present these details to the acting group at the end of the scene. Look for positive and negative aspects of etiquette to note among all participants.

1. Make two lists, recording "appropriate" etiquette observations in one list and "needs improvement" etiquette observations in the other.

_____

_____

_____

_____

2. Were any differences noted between the manners of the student-trainees and those of the employees? If not, should there have been any?

_____

_____

_____

_____

3. In a constructive manner, give your advice to the actors on how they can improve their etiquette. Reinforce the positive aspects you noticed.

_____

_____

_____

_____

_____

Readiness Checklist

_____ I understand the overall picture of how my manners or etiquette in the professional setting contribute to my professional demeanor.

_____ I have considered and recognize any changes I should make in my posture or demeanor.

_____ I understand the possible consequences of not appearing to have a positive attitude, confidence, and a noticeable interest in my field.

_____ I have considered ways in which I can improve my verbal manners.

_____ I have gauged my level of appropriate wording in general professional conversation and am aware of any challenges I need to overcome.

_____ I recognize the major distracting behaviors, and I have thought of ways to overcome those that may apply to me.

_____ I understand the guidelines for the use of personal portable electronic devices such as phones and tablets while on site.

_____ Concerning my use of social media, I am aware of the actions to avoid in order to demonstrate a "clean" personal image.

6

Communication and Developing Professional Relationships

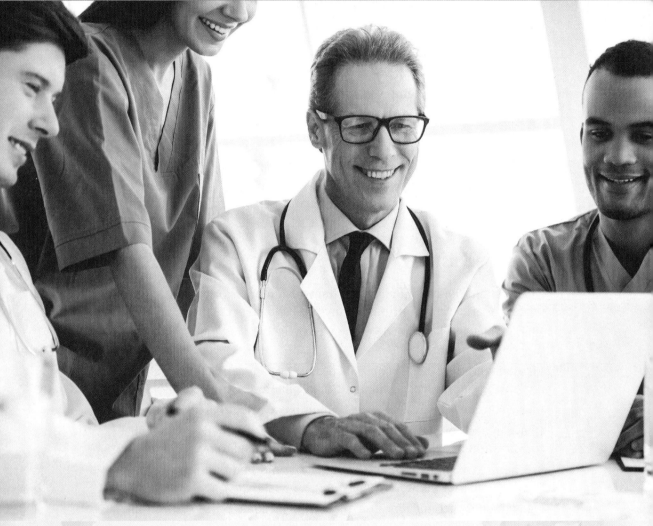

George Rudy/Shutterstock

The practicum is often the first opportunity students have to build relationships with established professionals in the field.

INTRODUCTION

This chapter presents the basic concepts of professional relationship development to keep in mind during the practicum. This will likely be your first real-world experience in the position for which you have been training. Although much more framework exists for fully developing professional relationships, this chapter is tailored to prepare allied health students for the most preliminary of these considerations for the practical training phase. The chapter concludes with Self-Prep Questions, a Role-Play Scenario, and a Readiness Checklist.

CHAPTER OBJECTIVES

- Identify five sets of skills that contribute to the development of professional relationships during the practicum.
- Describe the interdependence that exists among members of the health care team.
- Identify specific ways to initiate and develop healthy interpersonal relationships.
- Identify five examples of poor communication tactics.
- List three types of communication.
- List two key factors that help complete the communication process.

- Briefly describe what is meant by the terms *verbal*, *nonverbal*, and *written communication*.
- List at least twelve effective communication tips to practice during the practicum.
- Identify seven underlying causes of interpersonal conflict.
- Describe the meaning of conflict resolution and its benefits when handled successfully.
- Describe how to handle a personality clash in the workplace.

Building Professional Relationships

Your success as a professional depends greatly on your ability to effectively interact with other professionals. This involves fulfilling your role within the patient care team and avoiding or resolving difficult situations, such as personality conflicts that can affect your work. You should practice a specific set of skills in this area, including learning to be an effective team member, building healthy interpersonal relationships, using effective communication skills, resolving any interpersonal conflicts, and respecting the differences in personalities among your peers. During your practicum, tune in frequently to these aspects of professional relationships that define the working environment.

Spotlight on Medical Office and Facility Administrators/Department Heads

Within most allied health specialties lies the opportunity—to varying degrees—to advance into positions of management or administration. Although it is important to focus on building professional relationships in your specialty as soon as possible during your career, it is even more important to exercise this quality when aiming at advancing into positions of greater

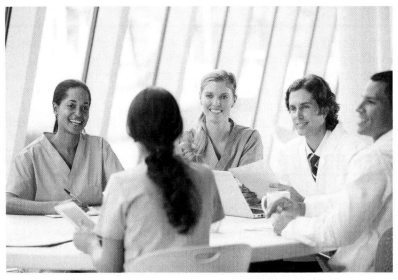

Teamwork, communication, and other aspects of interpersonal relationships contribute to the professional success of the student and medical office staff members.

responsibility, such as managing a department or a staff of health care professionals. Practicing effective communication and teamwork, working effectively with different personality types, and being resourceful in resolving any interpersonal conflicts are among the skills needed to succeed in such positions. When working in a leadership role, it becomes even more necessary to collaborate, promote a teamwork philosophy, and demonstrate interest in employee issues at hand and take timely action. Although it is always imperative to maintain excellence in the technical skills of your specialty, the relational aspect of working with your staff/team is important to becoming an effective leader in your facility or department.

Functioning as a Team Member

By the beginning of your practicum, you should understand that you are going to be part of a team. Although you may perceive yourself as an independent worker, it is important to realize the interdependence that exists among the various functional areas and departments of your practicum site, in that each staff member relies on the correct functioning of and the receipt of correct information from all other staff members. This includes all clinical and administrative staff. If you are a clinical trainee, your work as a medical assistant (MA), phlebotomist, X-ray technician, and so on will provide important information for patient management and all treatment prescribed by the doctor, physician assistant (PA), or nurse practitioner (NP).

After the clinical staff members visit the patient, complete specific tasks, and document them in the patient chart, those working with medical records, insurance billing, referrals, prescription and lab order phone calls, legal issues, and the like use these notes to complete the patient's visit and lay the groundwork for the entire cycle of care. All staff members, including janitors, maintenance personnel, information technology (IT) professionals, and any other behind-the-scenes laborers, are important contributors to the overall operation of the office or facility, and you should acknowledge this through your interaction with others working within the same team.

Building Interpersonal Relationships

Building good interpersonal relationships as early as possible during your practicum will help you significantly. You can initiate the development of such relationships by being willing to learn from and help others, demonstrating courteousness, and using effective communication skills. Many of the proactive measures you can take in this area are the active forms of the ideal attitudes presented in Chapter 4. For example, think back to the brief discussions presented on the positive attitude traits of pleasant service to others, appreciativeness, genuine caring, and persistent use of good manners. These coincide with learning from and helping others, as well as being courteous. Give a thank-you when someone reminds you where to find a piece of equipment. Lend a helping hand to a team member who might be behind schedule in his or her tasks. Also be helpful when interacting with patients and customers.

Communicating Effectively

There are entire textbooks, and even college degree programs, devoted to the subject of effective communication, as the topic is vast. This text presents a few basic points that you should remember specifically for your practicum, such as how communicating *effectively* influences your professional relationships positively. If you can achieve that skill, you will be in a position to say what you mean and to be understood by your listener or receiver as you intended. This enables you to avoid the consequences of poor communication, which can stall your learning and advancement in your field.

Among the numerous poor communication tactics you should avoid are blaming others, not thinking before you speak, talking too much, giving unsolicited and maybe even unwanted advice, and bragging, all of which will lead to undesirable results. Fortunately, all poor communication can be avoided with determination and practice.

The major types of communication are verbal, nonverbal, and written. Listening and feedback complete the effective communication process, and your capacity to listen effectively influences your overall communication effectiveness. Appropriate and meaningful feedback—a response you provide to others or that others provide you—is effective only when active listening is practiced.

Your actions, tone of voice, body language, and gestures all fall into the category of nonverbal communication. The words, statements, questions, and commands you actually speak all fall into the category of verbal communication. The way you express yourself in writing (wording, grammar, and spelling) falls into the category of written communication.

Within the communication process, especially that which takes place in health care among health care team members and between these individuals and their patients, it is also important to recognize the components of encoding and decoding messages. As you may have learned previously in your studies, the message sender/communicator must first encode the message he or she wishes to convey. This involves translating ideas, thoughts, or information into whichever communication medium is being used—that is, spoken words, written words, or any form of body language, gestures, and so on. In professional communication, special emphasis should be placed on ensuring that correct encoding of your intended message occurs. This, of course, is intended to ensure that the message or information being communicated can be correctly decoded by the person, professional, or patient on the receiving end. Decoding simply refers to the receiver's interpretation of the message, which is based on those aspects mentioned earlier that comprise any type of verbal or nonverbal communication. When communicating, be sure to give thought to how the receiver might interpret your message based on the various signals you might project, such as word choice, tone of voice, facial expression, and body language. When communicating in writing, word choice, punctuation, and appropriate grammar and spelling are your signals.

Others can gather much about you through the way you communicate. In addition, as an active participant in the communication process, you should be able to accurately comprehend and interpret the feedback you are given by others. Recall the interdependency of the health care team described previously in this chapter, and imagine how effective communication is required for proper team functioning with minimal communication-based breakdowns or mistakes.

The following subsections contain tips that are highly applicable during the allied health practicum for each area of communication, as well as in your communication with staff members, patients, and customers. If you feel you need more in-depth tips on the art of effective communication, seek additional resources from one of your instructors or a professional within the career services department at your college or school. Many resources are available on this topic.

VERBAL COMMUNICATION

The words you speak should be clear and easy to understand. Speak using complete sentences. If you are working in a noisy environment, speak louder, but do not shout. The same applies when speaking to patients or customers over the telephone. Because you will be working in an environment where patient information must remain confidential, you must practice caution in how you communicate certain information and to whom it is communicated.

NONVERBAL COMMUNICATION

Your posture, eye contact, facial expressions, tone, and overall professional demeanor contribute to the messages you communicate daily. Employ the following brief tips concerning these aspects of nonverbal cues:

- *Posture.* You should always try to maintain an upright posture (as opposed to slouching or rolling your shoulders down and forward). Recall the brief discussion concerning posture in Chapter 5 on the topic of etiquette.
- *Eye contact.* Make eye contact with anyone with whom you are communicating. Avoiding eye contact makes others feel unsure about your confidence in what you are doing or saying. Also, it is simply not polite to avoid making eye contact. Put on a smiling face, too.
- *Tone of voice.* Be sure that your voice conveys friendliness and not frustration. Work inevitably becomes frustrating at times, but it makes no sense to pass on this frustration to other workers and patients or customers. Falling into this trap creates friction in your work environment and may prompt customers or patients to complain.
- *Overall professional demeanor.* Consider your overall professional presentation as you communicate with others. Do you feel that others with whom you are communicating will perceive you as professional based on your appearance, gestures, and movements? And will they be able to clearly understand your communicated message in the midst of your unique mix of nonverbal cues?

Use these factors in positive ways to improve your customer service skills and demonstrate professionalism. Patients and customers can read your body language and are more comfortable in their interaction with allied health staff when they can interpret that you are a sincere, caring, and helpful MA, office staff member, billing representative, pharmacy technician, or other health care team member. On the other hand, it is also important and to your advantage to be able to interpret nonverbal cues from others, whether co-workers, patients, or customers.

WRITTEN COMMUNICATION

Because most of your written communication will pertain to patient information, it is extremely important to express all information accurately in writing. A special emphasis for the health care professional is the patient medical record, both paper-based and electronic formats. In patient charts, be sure to write the appropriate information in the proper section. Be certain that all words, numbers, and medical abbreviations are clearly legible, and use proper grammar, spelling, and punctuation. If you record the patient's chief complaint, for example, write clearly so that other team members (MAs, nurses, physicians, etc.) tending to the same patients will be correctly informed about the patient's explanation of symptoms or reason for the visit. For insurance, billing, and referral purposes, this supporting information must be accurate and easy to follow from the patient chart.

The same applies when working with electronic records. Consider all the possible parties within the health care system that may access a certain patient's health care information electronically. This information must be correctly entered with no errors. Unfortunately, there are instances where costly mistakes occur, even with the use of today's advanced EHR systems. For example, erroneous information might be documented when drop-down menus do not contain the exact information needed or when templates are not thorough enough to document all aspects of a patient's unique situation or condition. In such cases, it is necessary to add notes to account for any information that may not be part of the automated tools within the record. Always seek help from a team member or other practitioner if you are working in the records system and notice instances where relevant and/or important patient information should be noted. It will always be worth the time it takes to ensure this level of correctness, as the costs of incorrect or incomplete documentation can be great. Legal action against the practice or physician is a common result of medical mistakes, including those that are traced back to documentation errors. Medical staff and practitioners can lose their license to practice and ability to secure future employment in their profession if found to be legally negligent, insufficient, or incorrect in their patient records maintenance. Needless to say, excellent documentation practices should be a top priority for every health care professional.

LISTENING

Pay attention, and make it a habit. Focus on the message being delivered to you by the spoken or written words of the communicator. Tune in to the nonverbal aspects of any message. Your feedback to the communicator cannot be fully effective until you have understood his or her original message. Ask for clarification if you cannot fully comprehend the message. When interviewing or conversing with patients and customers, be sure you fully understand their complaints, descriptions of symptoms, questions about treatment options and medications, and inquiries about their medical records or billing statements.

FEEDBACK

Do you provide appropriate feedback to those who initiate communication with you? Listening is key to the ability of providing proper feedback. Feedback should be relevant and timely. Your feedback may be needed immediately or later. Provide it at the appropriate time.

Practice diligence when providing feedback to patients and customers. You must stay within your legal scope of practice when communicating and providing feedback to them.

EFFECTIVE COMMUNICATION WITHIN UNIQUE PATIENT SUBGROUPS

In today's health care environment, most practitioners and allied health professionals are frequently engaged in the care of unique patient subgroups, such as the elderly, those with varying disabilities, and those from different cultural backgrounds. When interacting with these patients, some specific aspects of communication should be considered and put into practice. This is an important part of providing quality patient care, creating a positive overall working practitioner–patient relationship, and demonstrating compassion and courtesy.

- The following are some general tips for communicating with elderly patients:
  - Generally, allow some extra time for interviewing, taking the patient's history, and all other aspects of the patient encounter. Don't make the patient feel rushed in any way as you are conversing and giving instructions, as this often translates into simply being impersonal and unconcerned.
  - Speak slowly and clearly, and if the patient is hearing impaired, carefully adjust your voice as needed to ensure he or she can hear you.
  - Be sure not to use medical jargon. Rather, speak in simple words, and make any take-home instructions as simple as possible.
  - Always allow the patient enough time to speak, ask if he or she has any questions, and make eye contact to let him or her know you are listening intently.
  - As always, use good manners and try to create a warm feeling during the visit, as this is usually important to elderly patients.
- The following are some general tips for communicating with patients with disabilities:
  - As was noted for the elderly, allow time for a longer office visit, making sure the patient does not feel rushed during his or her visit.
  - Be sure to face the patient, and even if the patient is accompanied by a caretaker, make eye contact primarily with the patient throughout your conversation. You can direct the conversation to the caretaker when the patient may not be following what you are saying or asking. When this occurs, always communicate to both individuals, as the patient is still the main focus of your conversation.
  - Keep the focus of the visit and conversation on the patient's chief complaint or reason for the visit, rather than thinking of the problem at hand in relation to the patient's disability. Keep in mind that illnesses and injuries unrelated to the patient's disability are common, and ensure that your conversation follows the chief complaint or reason for the visit.
  - During patient exams, explain to the patient what you are doing and why, and if needed and appropriate, clarify anything necessary by demonstrating it.
  - Give the patient the opportunity to discuss anything or ask any questions; ensure your full attention as he or she communicates to you. Respond by validating any concerns mentioned, and address

these as appropriate or let him or her know you will pass along the concern to the physician or practitioner for the appropriate response. Be sure the patient's concern receives follow-up.

- The following are some general tips for communicating with patients of other cultures:

  - Recognize that cultural heritage can heavily influence the way a patient views personal health and medical intervention and that in listening and speaking the patient can sense your awareness of this. Your awareness and openness set the stage for a more comfortable and productive visit.
  - Be sensitive to the patient's concerns and views. Even if you personally cannot relate to or agree with what the patient conveys concerning any aspect of his or her health or health care, always listen intently and be supportive of the patient's efforts to maintain health or overcome illness or injury.
  - During the time you spend with the patient, focus more on building a positive rapport and relationship than on apparent cultural differences.
  - It is okay, and even helpful, to ask the patient what specifics you and the health care team should understand regarding his or her cultural beliefs about personal medical care in order to best plan treatment, follow-up, and at-home care.
  - As with all patients, be respectful in all circumstances. Make it your goal for the patient (and the family) to know that you and the care team are truly concerned with and dedicated to the patient's health outcome regardless of beliefs, ethnicity, and cultural influences.

Issues of Conflict and Conflict Resolution

All students hope for a pleasant practicum experience. Occasionally, however, some students experience interpersonal conflict with others at their site. It is not surprising that these issues arise, even for the most likable and delightful persons.

Generally speaking, conflict in the workplace is inevitable at times. Personality clashes, differing values and perceptions, differing expectations and goals, ineffective communication, and competitiveness are all underlying causes. Most people see conflict as only bad; however, it also enables those who work through it diligently to reach resolution and experience personal and professional growth. The keys to a positive outcome are to recognize the onset of conflict before it causes anybody to compromise on the effectiveness of their work and to find a way to resolve the interpersonal issue at hand. This is often referred to as *conflict resolution*.

If you experience any interpersonal conflict while at your site, seek advice or help immediately. Do not be quick to verbalize questionable or negative thoughts about others, especially while at your site. Instead, contact your practicum coordinator and faculty regarding the issue. Be honest with the details of your personal perception of the problem, and consider any advice offered by your practicum coordinator or career services staff. Depending on the situation, the practicum coordinator may meet or speak with the site supervisor to discuss the issue and decide on an effective resolution.

Sometimes, the perception of one or more individuals is what causes an interpersonal problem. If this affects you during your practicum, take a proactive role in attempting to resolve the problem. Alternatively, you may ask "Couldn't I just be placed at a different training site?" The answer given to my students is "No" until we all have attempted to reach a resolution.

A resolution is usually possible if all parties choose to cooperate. If you run away from the issues, you forego a chance to gain experience that may be useful later in your career, and the same type of situation is likely to arise again.

If it arises, interpersonal conflict can be the most challenging aspect of the practicum. Working through it and overcoming it successfully will be a significant professional feat.

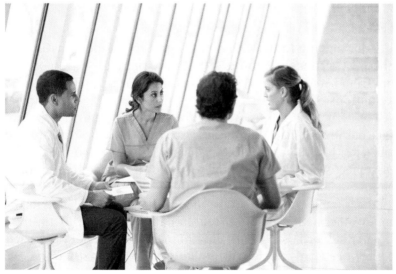

Shutterstock

Effectively resolving conflict requires cooperation and teamwork.

Overcoming Personality Clashes

Most people possess at least one personality aspect that you are not going to like. You probably have friends and family who have helped you realize this. What's important is to respect everyone's personality. If a quarrel with a friend or family member results from these differences, you typically have a good chance of reconciliation.

At your practicum site, when you realize people's personality imperfections and conceive your own opinions about them, do not let those opinions get in the way of your reasons for being at that facility or office. Do not let such personal irritations hinder your professionalism either. When others "get on your nerves," the best action you can take is to move, if possible, to a different area to do your work. Another option, which will take some mental effort on your part, is to focus on your reason for being where you are and achieving your goals of learning and succeeding in your practicum. Realize that you really don't have the time and energy to waste on others' irritating habits.

If the situation or annoyance becomes personal in any way or interferes with your performance, you may need to speak to your practicum coordinator and the site supervisor overseeing your work. On the other hand, remember that some of the people you are expected to work with may have opinions about *your* personality. Overlook personal annoyances and accomplish your goal of learning your specialty. Be realistic about the working world, expect that people will irritate you from time to time, and be empowered to overcome it.

Sexual Harassment in Today's Workplace

Beyond issues having to do with our abilities to get along with others and make the best of uncomfortable situations, there also are conflicts that result not from personality differences but from the inappropriate and unacceptable actions or behavior of an employee or manager toward another employee or even a student-trainee. Unfortunately, sexual harassment in the workplace has increasingly become an issue across all types of organizations and industries, health care included. Therefore, it is important to be aware of its existence, what it is, and how to report it if encountered during the practicum.

Sexual harassment includes unwanted and unwelcome behavior, communication, or other action that is sexual in nature and creates an uncomfortable, threatening, or hostile work environment. It does not necessarily have to be experienced only in person; it can be "virtual"—that is, it can take place through e-mail, texting, and other electronic means. General examples of sexual harassment include but are not limited to the following, all of which are unwelcome advances:

- Direct communication of a sexual nature, such as jokes, telling stories, asking questions

- Showing images with sexual content
- Gestures or other actions that are of a sexual nature

In any situation where a student-trainee feels that he or she is a victim of sexual harassment, the first action is to follow the procedure established by the site or facility for reporting cases of sexual harassment, which can usually be found in its policies and procedures manual. If this information is not immediately accessible, report the issue to your department or site supervisor or manager in a private setting. In addition, report the matter to the practicum coordinator/administrator for your academic program. The matter must then be handled according to the policies of each institution.

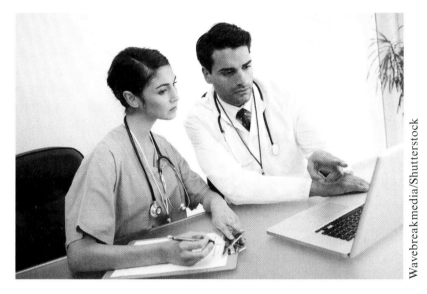

Wavebreakmedia/Shutterstock

Students work directly with health care professionals at the site; the result is not only gaining new knowledge, but also exercising communication skills on a professional level.

HIGHLIGHT

TIPS FROM PROFESSIONALS

I look for good work ethic and proactive thinking in the students I train. Students should make the most of their time, put forth their best effort and ask questions when needed. If down time occurs every now and then, the expectation is to be proactive and ask the manager what else you can do to help the staff.

–Office Manager (OBGYN practice)

Conclusion

In general, during the first few days of your practicum, look for ways in which you can be an asset to the team. Appreciate everyone's role in helping you learn, and make it a habit to lend a helping hand to others when you see the need. If along the way you are affected by any personal conflicts, ask for advice and seek to resolve them. When people's personalities or habits irritate you, do not take them personally; continue performing your work as a professional. Remembering and practicing these tactics will contribute to your overall level of professionalism.

Self-Prep Questions

1. Explain your role as an MA, administrative assistant, phlebotomist, X-ray tech, and so on in patient care. What will be your primary responsibilities? In what ways will you function interdependently with other professionals within the patient care team? (How will you depend on them, and how will they depend on you?)

_____

_____

_____

_____

_____

2. Recall the three major ways in which you communicate to others. Critique your own personal communication skills in these three areas, and identify the areas in which you may need to improve before your practicum.

_____

_____

_____

_____

_____

3. Briefly explain how listening and feedback are associated with effective communication.

_____

_____

_____

_____

_____

4. What actions would you take, and in what order, if you were to become involved in some type of interpersonal conflict while at your site?

_____

_____

_____

_____

_____

5. Explain what is meant by _sexual harassment_. Identify a few examples of behaviors or actions that illustrate this issue.

_____

_____

_____

_____

_____

Role-Play Scenario

Three individuals are needed for this scenario: the student-trainee, the office/facility manager, and the employee. The student-trainee has been given some tasks to complete by the facility or office manager. One of the regular employees at the site is instructed by the manager to supervise the student-trainee in completing these particular tasks for the remainder of the workday. This employee is normally the one who is working in the same area with the student-trainee, but today he or she has been assigned this supervisory role, and the manager has just recently mentioned to both the student-trainee and employee that this employee will be given the responsibility to supervise the student-trainee for the second half of his or her practicum.

Once the manager has instructed the student-trainee and has given responsibility to the employee to oversee the correct functioning of the student-trainee, the student-trainee begins to work diligently. The employee immediately lets this responsibility go to his or her head and turns it into a power trip. Although the student-trainee is performing satisfactorily, the employee is constantly finding ways to express his or her opinion and to correct things. The employee falls behind in his or her own work because of focusing on the student-trainee's work and looking for problems. Eventually, the student-trainee becomes fed up with this and approaches the office manager with the issue. The office manager must then propose a solution.

1. How should the student-trainee deal with the situation while still making an effort to finish the tasks on time?

_____

_____

_____

_____

_____

2. How long is long enough for the student-trainee to attempt working under these circumstances before he or she approaches the manager with the issue? Why do you think your proposed time frame is reasonable?

_____

_____

_____

_____

_____

3. How should the student-trainee communicate this complaint to the manager about the employee-supervisor assigned to oversee his or her work? Write out or verbally state specifically how the student-trainee should voice the complaint effectively and professionally.

_____

_____

_____

_____

_____

4. What are some possible solutions the facility manager could propose that might effectively address this situation?

_____

_____

_____

Readiness Checklist

_____ I understand the nature of my profession in that I am always functioning as part of a team: I depend on the work of others, and others depend on my work.

_____ I understand how to initiate healthy interpersonal relationships and that doing so boosts my level of professionalism.

_____ I realize that poor communication tactics have negative consequences. I have identified my tendencies in this area and will practice avoiding them for the sake of my success.

_____ I understand the importance of all three modes of communication in my career field.

_____ I realize that my listening skills are essential for the effectiveness of my overall communication.

_____ I realize the various aspects of people that may lead to interpersonal conflict in the workplace.

_____ I understand the importance of seeking a resolution to interpersonal conflict, and I understand that during the practicum it is important to seek help and advice from my faculty and site manager if a situation arises.

_____ I understand that people's personalities and habits may not be what I prefer. In such situations, it is best not to let these aspects hinder my professional work in any way.

_____ I understand that effective interpersonal skills are extremely valuable during my practicum, as well as in my future work.

_____ I understand the defining aspects of sexual harassment in the workplace and how to approach and report the issue if encountered at my practicum site.

_____ I understand how effective interpersonal skills contribute to my professional success.

7

Fulfilling the "Student" Role During the Practicum

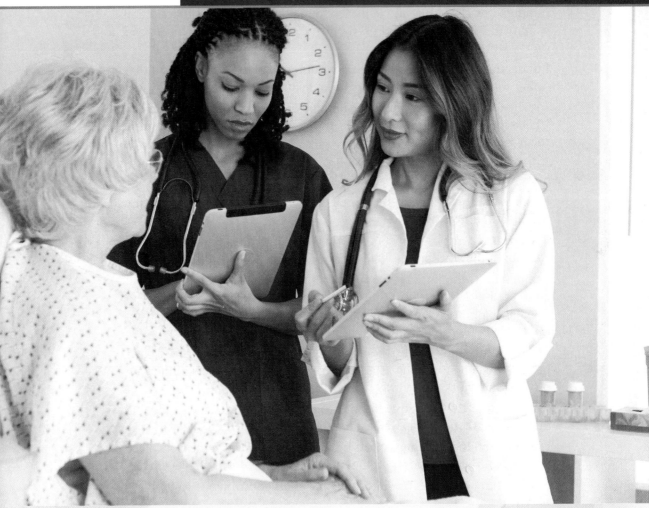

Rocketclips, Inc./Shutterstock

Fully engaging in the practicum requires proactive learning. This includes listening, asking appropriate questions, and taking notes.

INTRODUCTION

This chapter addresses the basic actions to be taken during your practicum for a successful experience. It describes how to be an active student-learner by being fully engaged in your work and taking initiative in your learning, while maintaining good student status. The chapter concludes with Self-Prep Questions, a Role-Play Scenario, and a Readiness Checklist.

CHAPTER OBJECTIVES

- Explain the importance of fully engaging in your practicum.
- Identify three benefits of fully engaging in the practical experience.
- Identify six examples of how to fully engage in your work at the practicum site.
- Identify three drawbacks of not fully engaging in the practicum experience.

- List six questions that will determine whether a student-trainee is fully engaged in the practicum.
- Name two ways in which the student-trainee is responsible to the supervising practicum faculty or coordinator.
- Name at least five types of information that should be recorded in your daily practicum notes or journal.

Fulfilling Your Responsibilities

To some students, the words *practicum, externship,* and/or *internship* imply not being in school. Although physically you will not be on your school's campus, your practicum site will become your temporary place of learning. Participation is mandatory, attendance is accounted for daily (as scheduled with the site), and the accumulation of your efforts and performance will earn you your final grade, just like any other course you have completed. Many students are motivated to begin this phase; a few tend to see it as a time to slack and, therefore, do not take their responsibilities seriously.

This is the trade-off: You are expected to become fully engaged in your profession and apply all that you have learned in the classroom while temporarily moving away from the type of learning that involves book work, classroom assignments, and exams. Thus, it is imperative that you perceive this phase as the most important part of your training. If you are thinking of slacking during your practicum, or you have not established a serious mindset, you risk losing control of your success, at least in the immediate future. Consider this seriously, keeping in mind that this is your first opportunity to earn a good reputation for yourself in your new career field.

Engaging in and Benefiting from Your Practicum

Fully engaging in your work every day is a necessity; there are priceless benefits in doing so. Remember: Nothing compares to the real-world portion of your training. Most disciplines of allied health are considered hands-on, intimate professions, and one benefit of full engagement in your practicum is perfecting or fine-tuning the technical skills you learned in the classroom.

No matter what your specialty is, daily practice of various tasks is essential for development of your practical skills. It is what you will be employed to do soon, so use this time to become more comfortable and efficient in your techniques. For example, a medical assistant (MA) practicum includes technical skills such as taking vitals and blood pressure, giving injections, performing EKGs and urine analysis, drawing blood, documenting or charting, and scheduling appointments.

Another aspect of full engagement is realizing the scope of what it means to work as part of a professional team (see Chapter 6). Reading about team dynamics is a helpful start, but the actual experience is a form of learning that you are more likely to retain. You will have the opportunity to observe the levels of interdependence that exist among allied health, nursing, physician, administrative, and business staff members.

The facility staff at your site will notice whether or not you are engaging in learning and applying yourself, and this can work for or against you, depending on your level of engagement. Their observations will definitely matter in your practicum evaluation and grade, and they could influence the start of your career. For example, staff at your site may be evaluating you discreetly for possible future employment, or they may be doing so for another office that may need to hire additional staff. You never know who is watching you or when. If you are fully engaged in your practicum, you will definitely begin your career with good rapport in some corner of the industry. This can help you tremendously in the future.

Following is a brief recap of the benefits of fully engaging in your work at the training site:

- Fine-tuning your technical skills
- Experiencing working as part of a professional health care team
- Earning a good or excellent practicum grade
- Developing good rapport with your site for professional reference in the industry

How to Engage in Your Work

To gain the most and best experience and knowledge, as well as to show your enthusiasm for the allied health profession, it is important to fully engage in your practicum. This may be done in a variety of ways:

- Ask questions
- Take notes or maintain a journal
- Be present
- Solicit feedback
- Offer your help
- Take initiative and assume responsibility

ASK QUESTIONS

You are a student, and the staff working with you will expect that you have questions or uncertainties every now and then—and more often in the first few days of your training—as you become familiar with the setup and daily operations at the site. Asking questions benefits you in ways other than just clarifying your uncertainty. For example, it shows the staff and site supervisor that you are interested in getting things done right and that you are respectful of adhering to the preferences of the staff, doctors, and so on.

TAKE NOTES OR MAINTAIN A JOURNAL

Good students take notes in class, and although you are not in a classroom during this phase, it is important that you treat the practicum as another class—that is, you should try to absorb as much new information and insight as possible. You might be required by your specific program of study to maintain a journal or compile daily notes as a course assignment. Documenting your experiences, new skills and techniques learned, and other general professional experiences in a journal or notebook is useful for personal reference or for any later project or writing assignment having to do with your practicum. It also demonstrates to the site staff and supervisor that you value their input and methods of training and that you are a responsible trainee.

BE PRESENT

With or without reason, some students find themselves slacking off when it comes to site attendance. However, the importance of attendance cannot be emphasized enough because you will not learn or progress without regular attendance and fulfillment of your commitment. Poor attendance also irritates and inconveniences site supervisors and trainers because it makes it impossible for them to complete their own plan for your training, and it affects the entire staff's dependence on you to fulfill certain, planned tasks. This is such a serious matter that your absence at scheduled times may result in you being dismissed permanently from the site. *Take your schedule seriously.*

SOLICIT FEEDBACK

Don't wait for the final evaluation at the end of the practicum to gauge your progress. Make it a point to ask your supervising staff trainer or manager each week for input on your performance. Ask what areas they think you need to improve on, whether your efficiency in getting tasks done is up to par, and how they would assess your professional development. Those training you will consider it very responsible and professional of you to ask these questions. Additionally, you will have ongoing (for the duration of your practicum) feedback with opportunities to improve as you progress through your training.

OFFER YOUR HELP

As many professional site supervisors would state, "Don't just sit there!" During a slow time at your practicum site (if this actually happens), do not be reactive—be proactive. If the time comes when you have run out of things to do or have completed your assigned tasks early, ask what else you can do to help. This is another way to get involved and learn about other areas of health care functioning that will be helpful to you in expanding your understanding of the whole health care process, thereby adding to your professional development.

TAKE INITIATIVE AND ASSUME RESPONSIBILITY

Make yourself the type of worker who is always active. Adopt the attitude that you have an important job to perform and people to serve. When problems or issues arise, think about possible solutions and ask others for assistance rather than leaving the issue alone simply because you are not an official employee. Help set up and clean up. If customers or patients are waiting to be greeted at the check-in desk, and no other employees are available at the moment, greet the customer or patient and state that the appropriate staff person will be available shortly. Adopting habits like these help you quickly develop into a productive and desirable worker.

The Problem of Disengagement

In significant ways, not engaging in your work daily has its drawbacks. First, if you are overly disengaged, your site supervisor may dismiss you permanently because staff trainers tend to view having such a student as a waste of time.

Second, community and regionally associated medical facility managers and administrators tend to know each other through professional organizations and affiliations, and they converse often. The last thing you should want is for your name to be associated with the label *Caution!* within your local professional community. The health care community is eager to praise those who work hard and go the extra mile, but recognition is also widespread for individuals who are regularly unproductive or have attendance or personal issues at work.

Third, your personal disengagement while at the practicum site is detrimental to your learning. If you are not active daily in taking on the challenges presented and learning from others, you are jeopardizing your own opportunity to gain everything mentioned in the previous paragraphs. Essentially, it would be a waste of time to go through the practicum without the will to learn and grow professionally. So, do the opposite: Engage in your learning.

The following briefly recaps the drawbacks of not fully engaging in your work at the practicum site:

- Probable dismissal from the site
- Beginning your career without the rapport you otherwise could have gained, and possibly creating a negative vibe that can spread through parts of the local health care community
- Wasting your time and the valuable opportunity to learn more for your own professional growth

How to be Fully Engaged

If you are reading this in advance of your practicum, use the following questions to prepare to be fully engaged in this learning experience. If you have already begun your practicum, use the following questions to determine if you are fully engaged in it:

- Do you attend your site as scheduled and arrive on time daily?
- Do you arrive prepared?
- Do you have a positive and helpful attitude every day?
- Do you ask appropriate questions to enhance your learning?
- Do you take notes or keep a journal?
- Do you attempt to learn about areas of office functioning other than those in which you typically work?

Spotlight on Paramedic and EMT Practicums

The very words *emergency medicine* convey a sense of high alertness, attention to detail, precision, and involvement. As EMTs and paramedics must be on their toes, so to speak, in responding to emergencies and in emergency transport, the practical training experience is a vital time within the training program for these student-trainees to focus and become fully engaged in applying lifesaving skills. The EMT can encounter any given medical emergency at any time and must be fully prepared and knowledgeable to provide care at that critical time. The practicum is an opportunity for experiencing these realistic cases for the first time. Active listening, mental clarity, and attention to detail must be practiced in order for these individuals to acquire maximal learning throughout their training and become fully functional and effective in their profession.

HIGHLIGHT

TIPS FROM PROFESSIONALS

In your training, remember that to make your best impression on the staff and providers, you must be professional in all aspects....timeliness, communication (especially if there is a time you are running late or cannot attend), initiative, and politeness to your co-workers and patients.

–Registered Nurse and Office Manager (Internal Medicine practice)

Acting Responsibly

To ensure that you are being a responsible student and fulfilling all of your practicum requirements, you should follow these steps:

- Maintain communication with your school.
- Maintain an academic or learning mind-set.
- Maintain proper procedures for absences and tardiness.

Maintaining Contact with Your School

Aside from the effort you put forth at your site, you have other responsibilities as a student. You must maintain active communication with your practicum coordinator and any other faculty or staff from your school involved in your practicum or program completion (financial aid office, registrar and student account offices, career services, etc.). You should note what contact is expected of you before beginning your site training. Your main contact obviously will be with your practicum coordinator or supervising faculty member. You will be responsible for providing a daily or weekly verifiable record of the hours attended. If proper information is not provided by you, you probably will not receive any credit for your attendance. Do not expect the site supervisor to be responsible for submitting your hours/time logs for you unless the arrangement between your school and the site manager requires this. If your assigned method of submitting hours is via fax, follow it up with a phone call to verify that it has been received. Likewise, if your assigned method is uploading the timesheet online and/or submitting it via e-mail, it is important to request confirmation of its receipt. Take initiative in these areas to maintain favorable student status with your college.

Maintaining an Academic Mind-set

Because you are technically still a student during the on-site training, you should envision yourself for the entire practicum in student mode, maintaining an academic mind-set. Realize early that this time will provide a significant learning experience. Just as you take notes in the classroom, you should take notes daily throughout the practicum. Keeping a daily journal may or may not be required by your academic program. Some programs require you to submit a final report on your practicum experience for a grade.

Whichever requirements apply to you, optimize your learning experience by recording a few notes daily about your experiences. A hidden benefit of doing this is that you can prepare for questions that may be asked of you during future employment interviews by reviewing these notes to vividly recall your experiences. Besides simply noting what happened and how to perform new procedures, make notes of what types of teamwork came into play, how you learned to communicate more effectively, and what strengths and weaknesses you discovered about yourself. Maximize your insights as much as possible for the sake of your personal and professional development.

Spotlight on Medical Assisting Certification

For MA students, preparing for either the CMA or RMA certification should begin around the final phases of the academic program or practicum. Depending on the accreditation of the school, the MA student will typically become eligible for either the Certified Medical Assistant (CMA) credential offered through the American Association of Medical Assistants (AAMA) professional organization, or the Registered Medical Assistant (RMA) credential offered through the American Medical Technologists (AMA) professional organization. If you are unsure of the certification for which you are or will be eligible, consult with your academic staff or program coordinator.

CMA (AAMA) students and graduates can apply for certification either near the end of their academic program, before graduation, or after graduation as either (1) a "recent graduate" (within 12 months of graduation) as a Category 1 applicant or (2) a nonrecent graduate (more than 12 months after graduation) as a Category 2 applicant. For current exam fees, refer to the AAMA Web site. Fees differ within some application categories based on membership status. The AAMA Web site also provides an Exam Content Outline and other valuable resources for refreshing your knowledge in advance of testing.

RMA (AMT) students and graduates can apply for certification based on meeting the requirements of one of the four qualifying routes for eligibility. For most applicants, eligibility will fall under the Education route. Students can apply before or after graduation with required academic documentation. For current exam fees, refer to the AMT Web site. Certification exam fees are not membership based. An online review of RMA exam content and a reference list are also available on the Web site, along with formal, detailed study resources that can be purchased.

Conclusion

The practicum is a new and completely different learning phase for you, but it is important to fully engage in learning while still a student and to equip yourself with all the knowledge you will need concerning your school's contact, attendance, and graduation processes. You will be off campus, and for some students it is very difficult to find the time to get back to campus once in the field for the practical phase. Be sure to speak to your immediate supervising faculty members to be sure that your expectations and vision are targeted correctly.

Self-Prep Questions

1. How do you plan to fully engage in your practicum experience? What aspects of your technical skills and professionalism are you seeking to exercise?

_____

_____

_____

_____

2. Do you know your school's protocol for submitting site hours? How often are time records due? How are the hours verified? What is the penalty for not following this protocol?

_____

_____

_____

_____

3. How are your school's attendance and tardiness policies applied to the practicum?

_____

_____

_____

_____

Role-Play Scenario

Two to four individuals are needed for this scenario. The student arrives at the office or facility as scheduled and finds that the office manager (no part to be played) will not be at the site today. The student has already been training with this staff for two weeks. Create a scene showing how the student can create a productive working day without the guidance of his or her usual site supervisor. (Other than the student, the other individuals participating should be regular employees who work in surrounding areas at the site, and they should follow the lead of the student.)

1. What are the initial steps the student can take when discovering his or her usual leader will not be available to assign and oversee tasks? (There are several options for appropriately handling this situation.)

   _____

   _____

   _____

   _____

   _____

2. How can the student devise a plan of action for the day?

   _____

   _____

   _____

   _____

3. Create a plan the student can work from to achieve a productive workday. Be sure to use time frames where appropriate for each in order to show effective time management in completing these tasks.

   _____

   _____

   _____

   _____

Readiness Checklist

_____ I understand the significance of fully engaging in the practicum.

_____ I understand the shift in my responsibilities in the change from classroom learning to off-campus learning.

_____ I am motivated to engage in and complete the practicum.

_____ I recognize the benefits of fully engaging in the practicum.

_____ I recognize the drawbacks of not fully engaging in the practicum.

_____ I understand how to determine whether I am fully engaged in learning at my practicum site.

_____ I am prepared to keep daily notes or a journal of my learning experiences during the practicum.

_____ I know my school's written requirements (if applicable) for completion of the practicum and how it will contribute to my grade.

_____ I understand that during the short-term practicum, I should not experience any tardiness or absences, unless an emergency situation arises.

_____ I know my institution's policies and procedures for tardiness and absences, and I have considered the fact that I will have to compensate for any time missed.

Benefits of Successful Practicum Completion

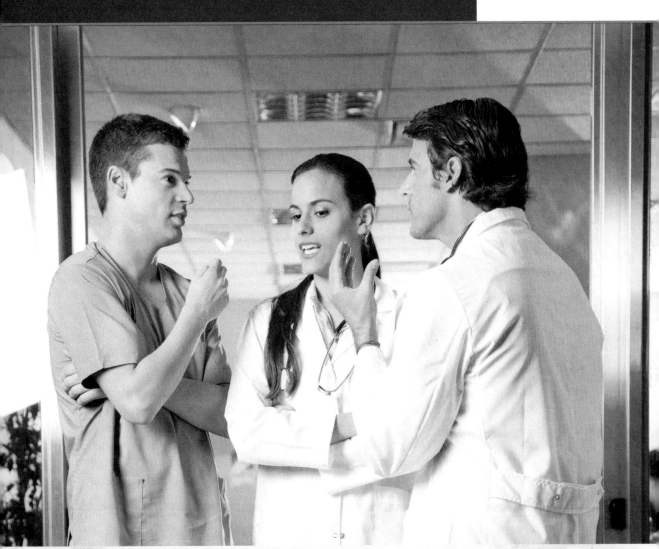

8

Tyler Olson/Shutterstock

An appropriate place to initiate your professional network is on site with your supervising staff members.

INTRODUCTION

In this chapter, you will gain insight into the personal and professional benefits that come with successfully completing the practicum. This chapter motivates allied health student-trainees to perform well in all aspects covered in previous chapters so that the maximum benefits available can be gained. These benefits include the fine-tuning of technical and people skills, documented practical experience in the new career field, new professional contacts and relationships, a beginning point for networking, at least one new professional reference, and possibly a job opportunity or direct link to one arising out of the practicum. The chapter concludes with Self-Prep Questions, a Role-Play Scenario, and a Readiness Checklist.

CHAPTER OBJECTIVES

- Explain the significance of the experience gained through the practicum.
- Identify actions you can take to maximize the experience gained during your practicum.
- Identify the factors surrounding the possibility of you becoming employed through the practical experience.
- Define networking, and explain how it can influence your career opportunities.
- Identify how to update your resumé with the details of your practical experience.
- Explain the importance of obtaining a professional reference from the manager or supervisor at the practicum site.

Your Entrance into the Field of Health Care

This chapter revisits the idea presented in Chapter 1 that your practicum is the *bridge* you must cross to advance from classroom work to the beginning of your new career. It is only after you complete the practical phase that you will be qualified with experience in an appropriate allied health setting. To emphasize the importance of the experience you will gain, it is typical that a medical office or other facility will prefer, or in some cases require, a certain amount of work experience in the field or your specialty as a condition of employment. Other preferences or qualifications, such as a specialty certification and proof of graduation from an approved program of study, may be required as well. However, these qualifications are on many occasions co-requisites to the level of experience required. In other words, your diploma or degree is not necessarily going to be seen by the health care community as a substitute for experience, so it is extremely important that you take full advantage of all aspects of experience offered to you by your practicum. Your connection to your chosen career begins in the practicum; it could very well be your opportunity to acquire a point of entry into the field in various ways, which is what this chapter discusses.

HIGHLIGHT

TIPS FROM PROFESSIONALS

The practicum process is so valuable to students because it provides the key to completion of the academic degree program, that "key" is experience. Experience provides students with the hands-on skills they may not necessarily learn in the classroom or lab, as well as the confidence that will help them excel in their first job. It doesn't end there, though. Learning takes place over the course of one's career, and making the most of learning opportunities impacts the individual's success.

–Practice Coordinator, Pediatrics Office

The Big Benefits

Following are just some of the benefits you will receive from successfully completing the practicum:

- Refining your skills
- Starting your career
- Networking
- Field experience
- References and letters of recommendation

Refining Your Skills

First, take full advantage of the opportunity to put your skills to work in the real-life setting of your practicum site. Fine-tune your skills and your ability to be versatile by being useful in many areas of the facility throughout the workday. Learn about as many areas as possible, even those that are not what you prefer to do most. For example, you may be a medical assistant (MA) who enjoys working one-on-one with patients in clinical procedures such as EKG and phlebotomy, but your practical experience should be balanced to include the full spectrum of clinical and administrative tasks. Remember that you are still in training and will eventually have the opportunity to seek out employment that is more focused on your preferred area of practice. The broader your experience is in the practicum, the greater the number of experiential skills you can claim later as professional experience. Not only should you learn as many techniques and practices as possible, but you should also pay attention each day to other areas, such as customer service, patient interaction, and team interaction. This type of learning is beneficial to you and may even help you to answer certain soft-skills types of questions as you interview for employment in the near future.

Career Launch Opportunities

Assuming you have performed according to all the rules and expectations of your practicum, you will have an opportunity either to become employed at the site or to obtain a strong referral for employment to another facility or office. If you develop a good working relationship with the team at your site, and the office manager is in need of an additional employee, you may be a favored candidate because you will have trained with the team already. Obviously, considering you for employment would imply that all your skills—your interactions with patients, technical skills, and reliability—are exceptional according to this team of professionals.

You have little control when it comes to being offered a job with your practicum site. Some offices engaged in training new allied health students are not in a growth phase and do not have the space or resources to add staff. However, the facility manager at your site may know that a branch location or an affiliated or neighboring office is in need of new MAs, phlebotomists, billing representatives, administrative staff, pharmacy technicians, and so on. What an opportunity that presents—and without the work of looking for vacant positions! Such opportunity has presented itself to many students who have put forth their best effort during the practicum, and a similar opportunity may arise for you.

Industry Networking

During your practicum, you definitely will have the opportunity to network with staff. This refers to you talking to various individuals and marketing yourself by building relationships and trust in your career field. Of course, you will begin your networking activities at the practicum site. As you gain experience and meet people from various parts of the industry, you will develop a unique network of individuals through whom you can seek opportunities. You can also inform those with whom you network about opportunities that may be suitable for them. The more people you know and have working relationships with, the more opportunities you will have access to while developing your career.

An easy place to begin your networking efforts, even before your practicum, is at your school. Your instructors, practicum coordinator, and especially your school's career services or job placement department may be able to recommend a few local starting points. Appropriate places to begin include, for example, on-campus career fairs and large-scale community- or citywide career events.

In today's world, it is important, and in many cases expected, that career-focused individuals represent themselves with an established profile within the LinkedIn online professional community. If you do not yet have a LinkedIn profile, this is an important task to complete in the immediate future. Your presence within this platform will enable you to begin networking online, a powerful addition to the networking you accomplish in person. You will be able to begin building your network with those individuals you already know from current or prior workplace experience, as well as those with whom you become well-acquainted through your practicum training experience. LinkedIn offers many features to help you market yourself professionally and continue to expand your network throughout your career. Further information regarding the uses and benefits of LinkedIn is discussed in Chapter 11.

Spotlight on Dental Assisting Practicums

Most dental assisting practicum students have the opportunity to network and make the most of new professional contacts at their sites. In group dental practices, a typical staff might include an office manager/administrator, two or more dentists and/or orthodontists, several dental hygienists, two or more dental assistants, plus a support staff of administrative professionals to handle patient records, scheduling, insurance and billing, and so on. This provides a number of opportunities for a dental assisting (DA) student-trainee to inquire about others' career experiences so far, to ask for professional advice in looking for positions, and to network in general. Some individuals employed at the site are likely to have contacts locally within the dental profession to assist a student-trainee in locating an initial DA position. The practicum site staff can be a valuable resource to students who will take this networking initiative.

Field Experience

Once you have completed your practicum, and before seeking interviewing opportunities, you should add the specifics of your practical experience to your professional resumé. This will enhance your marketability for the initial job search. Remember that your resumé should provide an accurate, professional, and positive image of you because employers usually will see this document before meeting you and learning about you. Refer to Chapter 11 for resumé-building tips.

The practicum is very useful when you want to include experience in the field on your resumé. List the name of the site, the beginning and end dates of your time there, and the total number of hours you completed for the practicum. Then list the duties in which you were trained and those you performed. Also include all the skills that you applied. Use proper terminology and spelling to describe everything. This section of the resumé is especially important to graduates who are entering the various allied health specialties for the first time. In addition, if you have volunteer experience in a related setting, be sure to include a full description, as this type of experience is also impressive to many professionals.

Professional Reference and Letter of Recommendation

Many employers seek professional references or letters of recommendation from job candidates. Through your practicum, you have the opportunity to acquire a letter of recommendation from your site supervisor and to ask that person if he or she will permit you to use his or her name as a professional reference. Do this completely at your discretion, but if you have worked well with the team members at your site and have maintained good, positive working relationships throughout your practicum, it is to your professional advantage to seize this opportunity.

Final Touches

On the last day of your practicum, do not leave without handing the site supervisor your resumé with correct contact information. If you were responsible for providing your resumé before the practicum, simply ask your supervisor if he or she would like another copy that includes the practical training experience you just completed. If your mentors at the site become aware of a job opening elsewhere for which they may refer you, you definitely will want them to have your most recent qualifications and contact information within reach.

If within a few months of your graduation you sit for and pass one of the credentialing or certification exams in your field, notify your practicum site supervisor of this by offering—in person—an appropriately updated resumé with this information. Each time you increase your professional qualifications, provide all your key networking acquaintances with the details, starting with your practicum site supervisor(s).

As a courtesy to those who have accommodated you at the site, it is highly recommended that you send a thank-you note or card to express your appreciation for their roles in helping you learn. Recognize them for taking time out from their schedules to help you and mention how valuable the experience was to your personal and professional growth. See Figure 8-1 ■ for an example of a brief thank-you note.

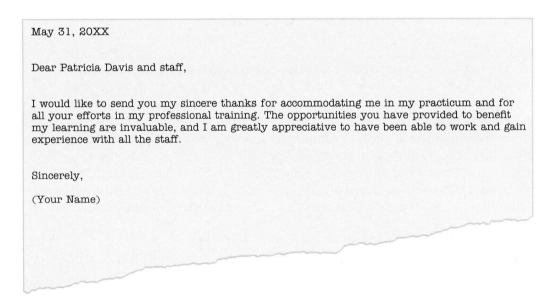

May 31, 20XX

Dear Patricia Davis and staff,

I would like to send you my sincere thanks for accommodating me in my practicum and for all your efforts in my professional training. The opportunities you have provided to benefit my learning are invaluable, and I am greatly appreciative to have been able to work and gain experience with all the staff.

Sincerely,

(Your Name)

Figure 8-1 ■ **Example of a thank-you note.**

Conclusion

As is apparent, you can reap numerous benefits from the effort you pour into your practicum. While still practicing the skills you learned in the classroom, you must have the mind-set that this practicum is really your first point of entry into your field and that many benefits are to be gained. Take advantage of the possibilities presented, and tailor them to suit your needs in gaining a professional edge.

Self-Prep Questions

1. Recall the benefits available to you through the practicum experience.

_____

_____

_____

_____

_____

2. What are some specific approaches to effective networking?

_____

_____

_____

_____

_____

3. Check the newspaper or Internet employment ads for your geographical area and your field of expertise. What variations are cited for the preferred experience or education level?

_____

_____

_____

_____

_____

Role-Play Scenario

Two individuals are needed for this scenario: the student-trainee and the office manager. Imagine you are a student who has completed your practicum hours; today was your last day with this site's staff and manager. *The scenario:* Your supervisor has planned a meeting time with you before you leave the site to review your performance and how you have progressed since the beginning of your practicum. For general purposes of this scenario, the supervisor gives positive feedback and is impressed with your performance. After this session, you initiate a brief discussion with the supervisor in an effort to begin professional networking for your upcoming job search. Prepare for how you will approach this opportunity ahead of time and what specific assistance you will request from your site supervisor in these search efforts.

1. What assistance will you request from your site supervisor? Be sure you are professional in making your requests.

_____

_____

_____

_____

_____

2. What plan will you establish for maintaining periodic contact with your site supervisor?

_____

_____

_____

_____

_____

Readiness Checklist

_____ I recognize that the practicum is a significant link between my classroom education and professional career.

_____ I understand that my documented work experiences are important considerations to my potential employer(s).

_____ I realize the opportunity and value in fine-tuning my skills, as well as building cross-functional skills.

_____ I realize that my practicum site is a valuable entity as it may likely become an important professional referral source or possibly a future place of employment.

_____ I understand that in order to expect a strong referral opportunity with the staff at my site, I must excel in applying my technical skills, interacting with patients and other staff members, and showing reliability.

_____ I understand that my practicum site can be a valuable first resource in my professional networking efforts.

_____ I plan to add the details of my practical experience to my resumé promptly on completion of my practicum.

_____ I understand the importance of updating my resumé, as well as my key networking contacts with this information, each time I enhance my professional qualifications.

9

Performance Evaluation and Your Grade

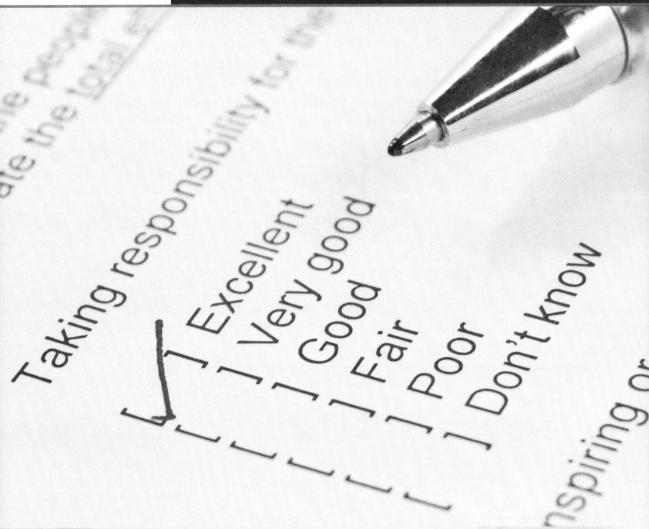

Mrfiza/Shutterstock

Your effort and performance determine the results of your practicum evaluation.

INTRODUCTION

This chapter summarizes the general areas in which most allied health student-trainees are evaluated on completion of the practicum. It presents straightforward explanations of the variations that are possible within evaluations, depending on which specialty of allied health you practice.

The areas of evaluation cover practical, clinical, and technical skills; administrative skills; and professional qualities. Beyond the evaluation given by the practicum site's monitoring supervisor, a few other requirements may contribute to your final practicum grade, such as a written report or other paperwork applicable to the experience. The chapter concludes with Self-Prep Questions, a Role-Play Scenario, and a Readiness Checklist.

CHAPTER OBJECTIVES

- Understand the nature of the practicum evaluation or grading process.
- Recognize the types of competencies included within each area of a practicum evaluation: practical, clinical, and technical skills; administrative skills; and professional competencies.
- View samples of practicum evaluation items for medical assisting and medical office administrative assisting.
- Identify several other possible requirements of the student for the end-of-term grade.
- Understand the content recommended for other possible course requirements.
- Identify various grading categories encompassing the practicum performance that can contribute to the final grade.

The Significance of Your Performance Evaluation

The overall goal of the practical phase of your education is to experience a set number of hours in a professional allied health environment in your specific area of study. However, it is important to remember that this phase is also a course requirement for which you will earn a grade. Your school normally maintains a syllabus or a guidelines document that defines the evaluation methods.

The way you are evaluated in your practicum is substantially different from the classroom grading criteria to which you are accustomed. This is a time when you have the opportunity to be taught and evaluated by a qualified professional of your chosen industry—a person other than your regular faculty. By the final phase of your practicum training, you should be looking for as much professional advice and constructive criticism as possible to help yourself prepare to enter the industry with confidence and reasonable expectations. Although you should perform to your highest potential, do not become frantic because you are going to be evaluated. You will find that the evaluation helps you to recognize your strengths more clearly and to identify areas in which you need improvement or extra practice. If you take these points seriously, especially the ones identifying your weakest abilities, and you do what is necessary to overcome them, you will be adding significantly to your professional development and value as an allied health professional.

The Basics of Evaluation

Various competencies for most allied health practicum evaluations can be classified into three broad categories: practical, technical, or clinical skills; administrative skills; and professional competencies. If you are practicing an allied health specialty with more specific skill sets (other than medical assisting and medical administrative/office assisting), your evaluation will not include the range of skills applicable to medical assistants (MAs) and medical administrative assistants (MAAs), as illustrated in the following examples, but it will include the set of skills for which you have been trained. Also, practicum skills and performance evaluations in some allied health programs can be divided into more specific categories or groups of competencies. If possible, at the beginning of your practicum request a list of the evaluation competencies in which you will be assessed. Familiarizing yourself with the focal points of your evaluation will help you define your professional tasks more clearly.

Medical Assisting Skills Evaluation

The following questions focus on competencies that are likely to be included in most MA student evaluations. Generally, the evaluator will rate your abilities on a given scale or will answer questions about whether or not you demonstrate competency in each of the skills or techniques listed. Questioning yourself concerning these skills before your practicum will help you notice areas in which you may need additional practice before beginning your on-site training. This is another proactive approach you can take for yourself to be better prepared for this training phase.

Professionalism, Career Development, and Readiness Competencies

- Do you show interest and intent to learn?
- Do you demonstrate critical thinking skills?
- Do you demonstrate attention to detail?
- Do you show empathy for all those you are serving?
- Do you follow professional ethical standards?
- Do you take initiative?
- Do you demonstrate flexibility or versatility?
- Do you adhere to the dress code?
- Do you have a clean and neat appearance?
- Do you use a systematic approach to problem solving?
- Do you demonstrate dependability (arriving to the site on time daily)?

- Do you show ability to organize work?
- Do you demonstrate effective time-management skills?
- Do you work as a team player?
- Do you work independently?
- Do you complete tasks on time?
- Do you demonstrate a positive, cooperative attitude?

Administrative Competencies

- How competent are you in efficiently handling correspondence?
- How competent are you in filing charts and other records?
- How competent are you in using effective communication skills?
- How competent are you in using proper telephone etiquette?
- How competent are you in greeting patients courteously?
- How competent are you in operating a computer?

Medical Assistant (MA) Practical and Clinical Competencies

- How competent are you in preparing patients for routine exams?
- How competent are you in assisting the physician or other practitioner during exams?
- How competent are you in maintaining the physical environment of exam rooms?
- How competent are you in assisting with routine eye exams?
- How competent are you in using medical and surgical asepsis?
- How competent are you in appropriately using personal protective equipment (PPE)?
- How competent are you in properly performing an EKG (electrocardiogram)?
- How competent are you in properly performing venipuncture?
- How competent are you in explaining treatments and procedures to patients?
- How competent are you in applying knowledge of sterile fields?
- How competent are you in administering medications appropriately?
- How competent are you in obtaining and recording vital signs properly?
- How competent are you in obtaining and documenting patient history appropriately?
- How competent are you in accurately documenting physical exam measurements and results?
- How competent are you in applying medical terminology?
- How competent are you in collecting and testing urine samples appropriately?
- How competent are you in applying documentation skills?
- How competent are you in using electronic health records?

- How competent are you in obtaining throat cultures?
- How competent are you in applying X-ray techniques and positioning? (If this is required of your profession, check state regulations for working with X-rays as requirements vary from state to state.)
- How competent are you in using lab slips properly?
- How competent are you in recognizing and practicing in accordance with Health Information Portability and Accountability Act (HIPAA) compliance standards?
- How competent are you in abiding by the legal and ethical standards of your practice?

Medical Administrative and Office Assisting Skills Evaluation

Another allied health discipline that covers a wide range of skills is medical administrative assisting. Students practicing in this area are evaluated in a number of competencies, including the full spectrum of tasks normally performed by administrative and office assistants in a medical facility. While remaining focused on providing quality customer service to patients, such students are primarily focused on the business aspects of the medical facility, such as maintaining records and paperwork, handling office phone calls and reception, scheduling appointments, processing insurance and payments, billing and coding, and so on. The following questions address the practical skills evaluated for a medical administrative assisting practicum. The professional and administrative skills listed in the preceding section are also applicable. Evaluations can instruct the evaluator to rate your abilities on a given scale or may question whether or not you demonstrate competency in each of the skills or techniques listed.

HIGHLIGHT

TIPS FROM PROFESSIONALS

In the MA practicum, students must recognize and become proficient in their roles in both clinical and administrative tasks. The experience enables the MA trainee to see the importance of his or her role as such in providing a complete patient visit, as well as general continuity of patient care over time. Some basics that MA students must be able to demonstrate during their site training are general math skills, as well as reading and writing skills. These skills support daily medical office tasks such as simple calculations, proper medical charting, correct spelling, and front desk competency.

–Medical Doctor/Pediatrics practice

Medical Administrative Assistant (MAA) Practical Skills

- Do you effectively coordinate patient appointments and scheduling?
- Do you demonstrate proficiency in collection and verification of patient insurance information?
- Do you submit insurance claims accurately and on time?
- Do you process patient payments accurately?
- Do you monitor reimbursement by third-party payers?
- Do you document accurately?
- Do you properly and efficiently file charts?
- Do you follow appropriate standards in helping maintain patient records?
- Do you correctly understand and use medical terminology?
- Do you understand and apply office policies and procedures?
- Do you use professional phone skills?
- Do you use professional communication in all forms of written correspondence?
- Do you understand and properly use diagnostic codes?
- Do you understand and properly use procedure codes?
- Do you recognize and practice in accordance with HIPAA compliance standards?
- Do you abide by the legal and ethical standards of your practice?

Learning from Evaluation Results

You may be evaluated in a wide range of areas. Educational institutions do not use identical evaluation methods or forms, but a comprehensive MA evaluation will contain the preceding major areas, with more or less variety. Typically, the MA would be rated for each of these competencies. Also, you may notice that the items in the Professionalism, Career Development, and Readiness category are those that are emphasized in this text. They are all significant features of your hands-on training and indicators of your overall level of professionalism. It is possible to conquer all the challenges of practical skills and administrative skills, but without professional abilities and attributes it is nearly impossible for one to succeed or maintain a good job record in any part of the allied health field. If you feel you are weak in these skills, do not be discouraged. Deciding to take steps to improve yourself in the appropriate areas and following through on a planned course of action will help you overcome any weaknesses and develop your professional attributes. Depending on the feedback you receive from your evaluation, seek assistance immediately from your instructors in any technical skills needing improvement, as well as from your school's practicum coordinator/faculty or career services/job placement assistance department in any professional skills in which you need improvement.

It is possible to do the practicum in a facility in which some of the listed clinical competencies are not applicable. For example, if the practicum takes place in a cardiology office, obtaining a throat culture, performing routine eye exams, and testing urine would not be applicable skills that would be evaluated in that setting. Likewise, the use of surgical asepsis skills would not apply in a family practice or general pediatrics office in most cases. Many evaluation forms typically allow for a *not applicable* (N/A) rating for instances such as these.

Spotlight on All Allied Health Specialties: Maintaining a Positive Mind-set through the Performance Evaluation

Many students, regardless of the program of study, become somewhat nervous concerning the evaluation of their practicum performance. This is natural, but students will feel more comfortable and perform better by understanding that their mentor/site supervisor is there to educate, support, and help. Yes, the manager/supervisor of the site will be the one to judge the student's performance; however, at the same time, this individual also willingly accepted the role of providing on-site training, development, and experience to the student. In most cases, students are trained and evaluated by professionals in the field who truly want to see them succeed. With this in mind, it is best to put aside any worry or negative stress concerning the evaluation process, simply take in the support and training offered, and continue working diligently for the duration of the practicum.

Other Practicum Completion Requirements

In addition to the practicum itself, many programs stipulate one or more other items that the student must complete. As noted in Chapter 7, two of the most common items are a daily journal to be submitted on completion of the required hours or an end-of-practicum written report. Another requirement that is often required is a practicum site evaluation in which the student has the opportunity to provide his or her personal and professional opinion about the site in which he or she trained. Know ahead of time about these student responsibilities by checking the practicum syllabus and communicating with your faculty/coordinator. More specifically, determine from your syllabus or by asking your instructors how these various end-of-term assignments are evaluated and how they will ultimately contribute to your final grade.

Journal of the Practical Experience

In assignments involving a journal (see Chapter 7), be sure to provide meaningful insights in the comments you record. Journal assignments may require somewhat brief and daily input or a weekly (or longer) more detailed account of your experiences. Unless you are given a specific format to follow, the most effective insight you can document is what new information or techniques and practical skills you learned, along with a summary list of the actual duties you performed for the given day. To go the extra mile in this effort, you may briefly record your experiences and outcomes in the areas of working as a team player, how effective or ineffective communication affected any situation, and how you may have gone beyond your assigned duties to help another (or how someone else did this for you).

Projects and Written Reports

End-of-term projects or written reports are most easily composed by those students who maintain a journal of their practicum experiences. At the same time, in the event of a relatively short duration practicum, many of the experiences will remain memorable enough to prepare the project or report immediately on completion of the required hours. Unless provided with a specific format to follow in writing a report, the following are several categories in which your experiences can be grouped to help you organize the experiences and insight you intend to present.

Topic Categories for Written Projects or Reports
- Briefly describe the personnel structure, type of facility, and medical specialty or specialties practiced at the facility.
- List all the skills you applied during the practicum.
- List new skills or techniques you learned that cross into other areas of the medical office or facility operations.
- Identify aspects of professionalism you were able to practice or enhance.
- Identify one or two instances in which conflict occurred within the team's functioning, and give your insight on the matter.
- Identify the most challenging aspect of your practicum.
- Identify the greatest benefit that you believe you gained through your practical experience.

Student Evaluation of the Practicum Experience

Many students are required to complete an evaluation of the practicum site. This allows the student to give feedback from his or her point of view as to the helpfulness of the staff trainers, the appropriate exposure to various profession-specific situations and tasks, and the opportunity given to apply relevant procedures and techniques and operate equipment. It also provides helpful information to the program faculty of the school, and it ultimately provides a benchmark reference for each facility's capacity to train students in various areas.

Grading

The final practicum grade is calculated based on the criteria provided to students in the respective practicum syllabus. Numerous factors can be used to determine the course grade. The following are several categories—but not all those possible—that can be evaluated and applied with a given weight toward the final grade:

- Professionalism
- Patient interaction and/or customer service
- Employee/team interaction
- Practical skills performance
- Written assignment(s)/journal/report
- Following instructions
- Time management
- Hours completed/attendance

Conclusion

The practicum will be evaluated on your performance in many attributes of professionalism, as well as on your performance, your skills, and objective measures such as written assignments. The practicum is your first opportunity to combine your best efforts in all areas of your prior training and to practice being a real allied health professional. Successful performance in all areas throughout the entire training phase will lead you to succeed in the practicum—and in the launch of your new career.

Self-Prep Questions

1. Identify the objectives/goal(s) of the practicum according to the course description given in your college catalog and/or course syllabus.

_____

_____

_____

_____

_____

2. Identify the method of practicum grade determination according to your course syllabus. (What categories are weighted together to determine your final grade?)

_____

_____

_____

_____

Role-Play Scenario

Two individuals, or groups of two, are needed for this scenario. The purpose of this activity is to become familiar with the evaluation form that will be provided to your practicum site supervisor and staff for feedback, as well as to understand how its results are formulated into a grade. One individual should act as the school's evaluating instructor/practicum coordinator; the other should act as the student. The acting student is to attend a brief meeting with the practicum coordinator to receive feedback given by the site supervisor with whom he or she has just finished the practicum. The practicum coordinator previously should have worked out the evaluation grade according to the school's scoring criteria. He or she discusses with the student the different skill sets evaluated and corresponding marks received and then explains how the evaluation grade has been calculated according to the syllabus.

1. According to your school's criteria, how are the scores classified and weighted to provide the final evaluation grade?

_____

_____

_____

_____

_____

2. How does this evaluation grade fit into the overall determination of the final practicum grade? What percentage of the grade does it comprise? What other requirements/grades will be weighted with this to determine the overall practicum grade?

_____

_____

_____

_____

_____

3. If your grades/evaluation results are less than you honestly expected, how would you respond to the practicum coordinator concerning these?

_____

_____

_____

_____

_____

Readiness Checklist

_____ I know the number of hours I am required to complete for my practicum, as stated in the course syllabus.

_____ I understand that a significant portion of my practicum grade will be determined based on the evaluation of my performance as judged by my site supervisor(s).

_____ I have discussed with my instructor(s) the set of skills in which I will be evaluated by the site supervisor, or I have viewed a document showing these.

_____ I understand the distinctions among the general categories of practical skills, administrative skills, and professional competencies.

_____ I am aware of all other course requirements I must fulfill in addition to the completion of the required hours.

_____ I am prepared to succeed in the practicum!

10

Allied Health Practicum:
Case Studies

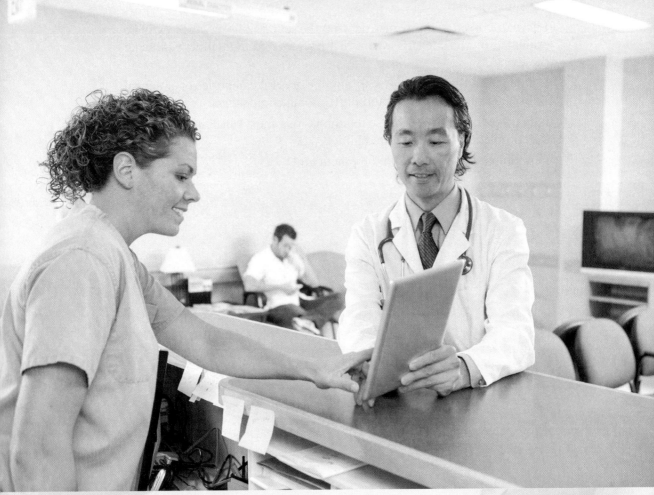

Tyler Olson/Shutterstock

Professionalism and preparation are required of students participating in the practicum.

INTRODUCTION

This chapter presents situations that have actually happened during student practical training experiences. The purpose of analyzing these cases is threefold: to reinforce the importance of the lessons presented previously in this text; to demonstrate the importance of true professionalism during the practicum; and, of course, to help all current and future students avoid the same mistakes. These scenarios reveal a wide range of areas for which the student must be fully prepared in order to begin the practical phase of training in a professional health care facility, pharmacy, billing office, lab, or other appropriate agency related to the provision of health care. These cases reinforce many aspects of professionalism, as well as areas of practical skills readiness. Each case is followed by a few questions to guide the student in examining its key components.

CHAPTER OBJECTIVES

- Examine various real-life scenarios of student practicum issues and dilemmas.
- Discuss the implications of the given situations.
- Provide possible solutions for improving the outcome of each case.

Case Studies

The following case studies are all real, but fictitious names are used to protect privacy. All practicum requirements and expectations were given to students when they entered the program of study, and these requirements are acknowledged by the students' own signatures required in practicum paperwork packets. Specific requirements and instructions were given to students before the start of the practicum, usually while students were in the final phase of coursework.

CASE STUDY 1: A DELAYED PRACTICUM

ALLIED HEALTH FIELD: MEDICAL ASSISTING

Allison was scheduled to begin the practicum in May. She was a medical assistant (MA) student. She had been out of school at least five months before the practicum but had previously completed all coursework necessary. She re-enrolled in school so she could complete the practicum and earn her diploma. When the time came for her to complete her pre-practicum paperwork and begin planning with the program coordinator, she could not be contacted at the phone number on file with the school. She did not answer or respond to any of the many messages left for her with regard to the urgency of her contacting the faculty by phone or visiting the campus.

A few weeks into the practicum term, she finally notified the faculty that she was ready to begin her site training. However, during the preceding weeks of no contact, she was dropped from the student body according to administrative policies. Obviously her practicum had to be postponed, and she was required to wait for the next term to begin.

While waiting, Allison received all the necessary paperwork and instructions for the required physical exam and TB test. Although she had a few weeks to complete these tasks, when she contacted the college to begin the practicum she still had not gone for a physical exam or TB test. Therefore, her re-entry for that term also was cancelled because of the lack of required documentation.

The practicum simply cannot be initiated without completed paperwork. Allison waited again for the next term to begin. By that time, she had completed the health documentation and was finally set to begin her practical training. All of this, beginning with the first re-enrollment attempt to complete the practicum, spanned four months—just to *begin* the practicum!

1. Give a brief analysis of the issues and problems involved in this case.

_____

_____

_____

_____

_____

2. Explain the measures the student should have taken and when in the context of this situation.

_____

_____

_____

_____

_____

CASE STUDY 2: ATTITUDES AND IMPRESSIONS

ALLIED HEALTH FIELD: HEALTH INFORMATION TECHNOLOGY AND MEDICAL ADMINISTRATIVE ASSISTING

Ryan was in the process of fulfilling his practical training hours in an internal medicine office. His programs of study were health information technology and office administrative assisting. Ryan's site supervisors had established a methodology of training throughout all areas of the office pertinent to his educational training.

The first area of the practical experience arranged was working with patient files, paperwork, appointments, and light correspondence. After the first two weeks of a part-time practicum schedule, and having already missed two days of attendance, Ryan began to show the attitude that he was above and beyond this level of training, although he had never worked in a physician's office before. His idea was that he would go straight to the billing and coding area of the office, which was actually planned for the final phase of his practicum by his site manager. As his "too good for this" attitude increased by the day, and as the professionals working with him took notice, the office manager finally contacted his college to inform the faculty of the attitude issues and that the office staff would no longer accommodate him. Therefore, Ryan suddenly found himself without a training site.

The practicum coordinator arranged a possible replacement site for Ryan, which required an interview. The interview time was agreed to by all parties four days in advance for 11:00 a.m. on the following Monday morning. On the day of the interview, Ryan showed up for the interview at noon—and without a resumé. The site supervisor, who happened to be the owner of the company, conducted a brief interview with him. For obvious reasons, the owner did not view him as a fit candidate for a practicum at that office. Therefore, Ryan was again without a site.

So far, one week had lapsed since Ryan had earned any practicum site hours or credit. A few days later, he was scheduled to meet with the office manager of a third possible site. He arrived on time with his resumé for this appointment, and after a brief interview he was accepted to begin his practicum the following week. (This delay is normal, as many site managers need some time to arrange to accommodate a student.) By the time Ryan was able to begin earning practicum credit again, he was in severe danger of being dropped from his program because of nonattendance. Only through the persistence of the faculty and college administration were a few grace days allowed for him. Ryan completed the practicum within a few weeks, but he did so with habitual complaints and imperfect attendance because of personal issues.

1. Give a brief analysis of the issues and problems in this case.

_____

_____

_____

_____

_____

2. Describe what cooperation was needed from Ryan during his time at the first practicum site. What benefits would have resulted from this? What differences in the outcome of his practicum would have resulted?

_____

_____

_____

_____

_____

3. State briefly the lessons that can be learned from this case.

_____

_____

_____

_____

_____

CASE STUDY 3: NO SHOW, NO SITE

HEALTH FIELD: PHARMACY TECHNICIAN

Ashton was scheduled to begin his practicum on Wednesday morning at 9:00 a.m. On Wednesday, the manager of the training site called the practicum coordinator to report that Ashton did not show up and had not contacted the staff. The practicum coordinator then contacted the student to ask why he was not in attendance. Ashton's explanation was "I did not go to my site this morning because something I ate last night did not agree with me, and I have not been feeling well. Late at night I needed to take medicine so that I could sleep. I was supposed to be at my site at 9:00 a.m. today. What do I do?" The student and the practicum coordinator both called the site, and fortunately the site manager was willing to issue a "grace" day in this situation and allowed Ashton to start on Thursday morning at 9:00 a.m. During this session, Ashton was reoriented by the pharmacy manager about the importance of daily attendance and professionalism, and this was reiterated by the college faculty as well.

The following Monday, the practicum coordinator received another telephone call from the site manager with the report that Ashton again had not shown up or contacted the staff. This time the manager stated that this was the final chance and that the student would need to complete his practical training at another site. The practicum coordinator contacted Ashton regarding this incident, and he reported the following: "I'm so sorry. I overslept. Nobody woke me up this morning. My cell phone alarm was set, but it was underneath my pillow, and I didn't hear it." Ashton was then informed that he had lost his site assignment, that he would have to wait until another one could be arranged, and that he would need to urgently and actively participate in the site search in order to expedite the process. More than a week passed before Ashton was able to resume his practicum at another site.

1. Give a brief analysis of the problems and issues in this case.

_____

_____

_____

_____

_____

2. Suggest basic measures this student should have taken to prevent this unnecessary pitfall.

_____

_____

_____

_____

_____

3. If you were the site manager in this case, what inferences about Ashton would you make concerning his repeated negligence in contacting the office?

_____

_____

_____

_____

_____

4. If you were a manager of a health care facility, would you refer this student to another facility or office for an employment interview? Think about how this pitfall will automatically give a student a negative reputation professionally, as well as what losses to the student may result.

_____

_____

_____

_____

_____

CASE STUDY 4: CONFIDENTIALITY BREACH

ALLIED HEALTH FIELD: MEDICAL OFFICE ADMINISTRATION

Shalane began her practicum in a medical office to train in the specialty of medical office administration. In the beginning, she received high ratings from her supervisors. They usually gave positive feedback concerning her attitude, performance, and professionalism. Several weeks passed before her practicum coordinator was surprised to receive a phone call during which he learned that Shalane had crossed a major line both legally and ethically.

The report was given that an acquaintance of a close friend visited the office with his spouse for an appointment to receive psychiatric evaluation and consultation. Apparently, the student said "Hello, how are you doing?" to this acquaintance, just to be friendly. The specifics of what happened out of the office are not clearly known. However, the patient (spouse of the student's acquaintance) visited the office shortly thereafter to complain that an office worker had spread the word that she had consulted with a psychiatrist for some reason. The patient told her physician that she had received information from a friend regarding the news of her office visit. In summary, this private information had come back to the patient through others whom she had never informed of this personal event. The information allegedly was initiated by Shalane, the student-trainee, who was the only person in the office remotely acquainted with the couple.

Because of this incident, Shalane was no longer allowed to participate in the practicum in this office. Not only did she suffer consequences, but it also hurt the possible opportunity for future students because the physicians and office manager made the decision that no students would ever be allowed again in that role in their practice.

1. What violation was committed by this student-trainee?

_____

_____

_____

_____

_____

2. What are the possible consequences not mentioned in the case that could have arisen at a later time for Shalane?

_____

_____

_____

_____

_____

3. What were the consequences to Shalane's school and fellow students, including future student-trainees?

_____

_____

_____

_____

_____

CASE STUDY 5: THE "A" THAT SLIPPED AWAY

ALLIED HEALTH FIELD: SURGICAL TECHNOLOGY

Justin was challenged to meet the minimum hours required each week for his practicum. However, he persevered throughout the practicum phase and met the expectation in this area. On completion of his practical training, he was required to submit several documents, including an evaluation by the site manager and several assignments regarding the practicum experience. The following specific items were required and outlined in the practicum syllabus as follows: evaluation by site (25% of final grade), student's evaluation of the site with short essay (25% of grade), journal of daily activities (25% of grade), and completion of all hours required (25% of grade).

Justin's evaluation by the site was submitted on time, and his score provided by the site manager reflected excellence in all areas, encompassing professionalism and practical skills in surgical assisting procedures and techniques. Justin opted to submit his journal weekly with his timesheets, so this requirement was fully met also. He completed the total hours in the time stipulated by the college, and this requirement was fully met as well. Several days after the completion of Justin's practicum, the college faculty and practicum coordinator were still awaiting submission of his evaluation of the site with essay documents that would be assessed for the final 25% of his grade. After several days of attempted phone calls to the student, it was finally concluded that his phone was out of service. The school sent Justin an e-mail regarding this final required assignment, but no response was received to this outreach either. When the grade for the practicum term was due to the college registrar's office, Justin's final grade was calculated based on the items completed.

Justin's grade was a C (75%) because he earned 0% for a component of the grade worth 25%. Even with a perfect evaluation by his site supervisor, his neglect in submitting the final assignment dropped his grade from a potential A (100%) to a C (75%). This is a drastic difference between what the grade actually was and what it could have been. This also negatively impacted Justin's final overall GPA. (Note: Many schools stipulate a minimum grade of C in the practicum as a graduation requirement.)

1. What are the simple steps Justin could have taken to prevent this major deduction from his final grade for the practicum?

_____

_____

_____

_____

_____

2. Explain why understanding the syllabus guidelines for grading the practicum is so important.

_____

_____

_____

_____

_____

CASE STUDY 6: SKILLS REVIVAL

ALLIED HEALTH FIELD: MEDICAL ASSISTING

Kara was set to begin her medical assisting practicum at a family practice facility. Before the practicum, she responsibly submitted all the required paperwork on time. Also, she excelled in the faculty-administered skills evaluation required before her practicum. Kara was even approved by her instructor while in the final phase of course-work to assist new students in learning how to read blood pressure.

Kara began the practicum with high expectations by her faculty because of her excellent performance throughout all her courses. Within two weeks of beginning the practicum, Kara's site supervisor notified the practicum coordinator that Kara did not seem to be competent in her skills, specifically blood pressure reading, venipuncture, and injections. It was also reported that Kara seemed exceedingly shy around the patients and staff. In addition, she did not exhibit any initiative to inquire about what she should be doing and for the most part was waiting for a staff member to give her step-by-step instructions on what task to complete next. The site supervisor stated that Kara did not seem like she had the ability to function on her own as an MA in an office or another facility. She also recommended that Kara return to the school for a brief review with the faculty before returning to the site. The site supervisor had good intentions in advising this as she did wish for Kara to perform well, demonstrate her competency, and become a qualified MA.

The staff at this office communicated what it thought would be the best route for improvement based on their work with Kara. They hoped they would be able to truthfully provide good marks or ratings for her final evaluation.

Kara returned to her school and worked with several faculty members on various skills for a couple of days. After a complete hands-on skills evaluation, Kara was again deemed competent in all clinical skills applicable to medical assisting. When Kara inquired about specific aspects of her interaction and fitting in at the site, one instructor advised her in the area of taking initiative, smiling and appearing pleasant, being assertive rather than acting shy, being relaxed rather than nervous in her venipuncture and injection procedures, and taking charge of her role now that she had learned how the office functioned. (All these specifics are very relevant to how professionals at a practicum site perceive the abilities and professionalism of student-trainees.)

Kara returned to her site with these key points in mind. Several days after her return to the site, the supervisor and other staff reported that Kara was performing much better, seemed more interested in her work, and was communicating much more effectively with the patients and staff. Because she was taking more of a proactive role in her work, she was able to work more in the lab. She also had opportunities to prove her injection skills to another MA, and was then allowed to perform several venipuncture procedures with patients.

Kara also was proactive in requesting that another MA work with her on using the type of sphygmomanometer native to the facility's patient rooms. She proved her mastery of this skill as well. According to her evaluation by the site staff, Kara completed the practicum with a good-to-excellent outcome—that is, of the categories scored, all were marked with ratings of "good" or "excellent."

1. What practicum outcome was likely to have resulted if Kara had not taken the advice from her instructor to be assertive, take initiative, and so on when she returned to the site?

_____

_____

_____

_____

_____

2. Explain how a lack of initiative and assertiveness could send the message to a site supervisor or staff member that a student is not satisfactorily competent.

_____

_____

_____

_____

_____

HIGHLIGHT

TIPS FROM PROFESSIONALS

I have been working with student-trainees in our office for a number of years, and based on these experiences, I have several recommendations. First is to be positive and use good communication skills, this is important when working with patients. It won't work out if you cannot communicate with patients and their family members. Another point is to make sure you are competent in your hands-on skills before you begin the practicum. We have had several MA students in the past that could not perform blood pressures and a few other core skills, which posed an inconvenience being that our office is quite busy daily. Your site manager will expect that you are already proficient in your skills, so be prepared. A final recommendation is to be as professional in your practicum as you would in a paid position, especially when it comes to your attendance and being on-time. If there are any days you are sick or late, it is expected that you call in to your site as you would a regular job.

–Office Manager, Family Medicine Practice

Beyond the Practicum: Beginning Your Job Search

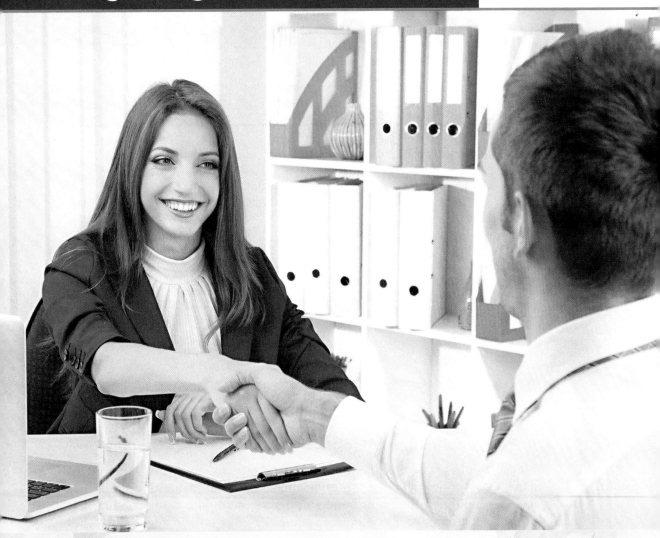

Africa Studio/Shutterstock

A professional image, both in person and on paper, is essential to successfully progressing through the job search, application, and interview processes.

INTRODUCTION

This chapter introduces the basic steps to be followed in the process of the job search. It blends general expectations with various specialized aspects for allied health job searches. Student-trainees should begin the preliminary steps of this phase during the practicum, if possible, or immediately upon completion of the practicum, unless further education or coursework is to be completed before that. The topics covered include becoming familiar with local job markets, writing resumés and cover letters, preparing for a successful interview, and following up on interviews with thank-you letters. To optimize the job search, it is highly recommended that, in conjunction with using this guide, you work closely with your career resource center on campus if available.

CHAPTER OBJECTIVES

- Identify resources for becoming familiar with the local job market.
- Describe the goal of an effective resumé.
- Identify and compare the four basic resumé formats.
- Define *transferable skills* and give examples.
- Describe and identify an effective entry-level resumé.
- Identify specific allied health qualifications that should be included in the resumé.
- Describe appropriate formatting for building the resumé.
- Describe appropriate writing for building the resumé.
- Explain the overall goal of the cover letter.
- Describe how to accomplish the goal of the cover letter.
- Describe the process of applying for jobs online.
- Explain the importance of appropriate voice-mail messages and e-mail addresses for professional correspondence.
- Describe the proper attire and appearance for an interview.
- List the issues of etiquette to be followed for the interview process.
- Describe appropriate preparation for phone and video interviews.
- Describe the goal and the main contents of the thank-you letter.

A Process with Many Steps

Multiple steps are involved in the job-seeking process, and you can put forth much effort to improve your interviewing skills. The earliest search phase includes building your resumé and gaining a general idea of the job market in your geographic region. Consider going the extra mile by researching the companies or medical practices in which you are interested before the interview; this will prepare you to ask intelligent questions of interviewers. Other considerations include writing and submitting a catchy cover letter with your resumé and then writing a sincere thank-you letter to all subsequent interviewers. Practicing professional etiquette and dressing appropriately for the interview are also important, as interviewers form their first impressions of you based on your actions and appearance.

All your efforts in these areas will prove significant as you strive to secure a position you desire. In general, taking a proactive approach to your job search will provide you with the best results.

Becoming Familiar with the Local Job Market

Gaining familiarity with the job market in your area is a process that requires time and a diligent search, beginning with the fact that employers advertise job openings in many ways. Although it is quite easy to use various Internet job and career sites to find advertised positions, this will never provide an adequate picture of the available jobs in a given city or region. Also, Internet methods of collecting resumés are more likely to be limited to "collecting." Some companies do maintain their Internet postings simply to collect resumés without actually having an immediate need for employees. This is not meant to discourage anyone from searching within these Web sites. The job descriptions and salary information, if noted, provide useful information for all who seek employment. In addition to job sites on the Internet, refer to the listings of jobs by category in local newspapers. These sources are likely to contain postings by local organizations for positions that are somewhat immediate. Respond to ads for positions listed in local sources within a day or two of the posting. Check the same source as often as it is updated, and you will begin to gain familiarity with the demand for certain jobs within allied health, the minimum qualifications and experience required, and possibly the salary range, although some companies choose not to publicize their salary information.

Other approaches to job searching may require more time and effort. If you are interested in certain companies, hospitals, or health care systems, go directly to the Web sites of these organizations. A link to "Jobs," "Employment," "Human Resources," "Careers," or some other related page is usually accessible from the organization's home page and will lead you to a listing of available positions. Large organizations' Web sites will typically include a job search page with search filters, enabling job seekers to view vacancies by position type, title, and location.

Various actions will then be required of you, the applicant. Many organizations have an online electronic application that prospective candidates must complete, and very likely a designated field in which you are to copy and paste or upload your resumé. Anytime a resumé is to be submitted online, be sure that the font is one of the basic types and that no graphics, word art, and the like are present. It will be helpful to create and store a second resumé specifically for electronic submission, especially if your original resumé contains bullets or fonts that can change during electronic submission. When your application is submitted directly through a company's Web site, it is important to take time to complete the application in its entirety, emphasizing your marketable qualifications in the appropriate areas. Always proofread the electronic application before submission.

Other resources that may be available through your school are the on-campus career services, career resources, and job placement offices. The people working in these offices generally have a working knowledge of the latest job opportunities and areas of employment growth within the local communities, and they generally provide students and graduates with assistance for creating and updating their resumés, writing their cover letters and thank-you letters, and learning about successful interviewing. Most also have ongoing relationships with various employers, which can be very helpful to graduates of allied health programs.

Another great opportunity for students and graduates is to keep abreast of the schedule of various job fairs that take place within local and nearby communities. Information for these events can typically be found online at various job Web sites, on local TV news coverage, on radio commercials, and from career assistance offices. It is beneficial to attend these events while you are still a student and to present yourself professionally: Wear clothing appropriate for interviewing and carry a professional-looking organizer large enough to hold at least 10 unfolded copies of your resumé. At these events, employers seek to collect resumés from job candidates and, sometimes, to perform on-the-spot interviewing and hiring. By the time you attend this type of event, perfect your interview techniques and other formalities, such as a firm handshake and professional introduction of yourself, so you can make a very positive first impression on potential employers.

Depending on the outcome of your practicum experience and whether or not a good relationship was built with the site manager and staff, you can network with previous trainers and mentors about job openings in their facility or other facilities with which they are affiliated or acquainted. Provided that a very good-to-excellent practicum experience took place, the staff from the site will likely be able and willing to give your name and a good recommendation to their peers. Try to maintain this level of relationship with your practicum site staff for at least a few years. If feasible, always provide the staff at the site with a periodic update of your experience and increasing qualifications.

Whichever combination of these resources are used to begin the job search, you are advised to be as proactive as possible when researching the local job market. Those who have the assumption that their school or college is responsible for their employment, even when job placement assistance is provided by the institution, lose many opportunities that they may otherwise discover for themselves by networking and using additional methods. The career assistance offices within schools are valuable resources, especially for students and graduates without experience in the job-seeking process; however, the services they provide should be accompanied by your own search efforts to maximize opportunities. Motivation is key in this process, and the motivating factor is that the amount of effort put forth in the job search will provide a proportional amount of opportunities for interviews and employment options.

The benefits gained by taking a proactive approach are as follows.

- You can see for yourself what the trends are in minimum qualifications.
- You can recognize a group of effective key words relevant to the field in which you are seeking employment (useful in resumés and cover letters).
- You can use various resources to keep abreast of industry demands.

Resumés

This section introduces three basic types of resumés, some valuable resumé tips, and sample resumés. The main concept to recognize in building an effective resumé is that it must paint a clear, realistic, and desirable picture of the professional *you*. It must reflect the totality of your accomplishments and professional experiences.

Essentially, your resumé is your application for an interview. Think of the moment when a potential employer is looking through a stack of twenty-five resumés, one of which is yours. How will you ensure that yours will stand out among the others? Those selected for interviews will have presented the most appropriate, impressive, and easy-to-follow resumés, with the required minimum skills, education, and other qualifications, of course. Selecting the most appropriate resumé format conducive to your work history, experiences, and education will provide the best picture of you. Using a style that is appealing will also tempt the reader to take a moment to peruse the entire content of your resumé. Organized headings with impressive, but not overdone, wording will also hold the reader's attention. While attempting to impress, it is important not to exaggerate content, wording, and design to the point where the resumé becomes gaudy, wordy, ambiguous, or difficult to follow.

The following sections will guide you through the basics of building a resumé.

Choosing an Appropriate Resumé Format

In building a resumé, you should consider certain aspects of your educational and work history before deciding which resumé format to follow. If you already have a resumé, use the following information to evaluate whether you have your personal work history presented optimally for your career goal. Several types of resumé can be used, and every individual should attempt to maximize his or her chances of obtaining an interview or becoming hired (or even chances of being accepted for the practicum). The four main types of resumés are the chronological resumé, the functional resumé, the combination resumé, and the entry-level resumé. Table 11-1 ▓ provides a brief overview of the suggested use for each.

THE CHRONOLOGICAL RESUMÉ

The chronological resumé presents the candidate's experiences in reverse chronological order. The work experience is listed beginning with most recent

Table 11-1 ■ Summary of Resumé Types and Suggested Use

Type of Resumé	When to Use This Format
Chronological	• To demonstrate a long, solid work history with minimal gaps between jobs • To reflect consistency, continuity, and growth or progression within a professional field
Functional	• To highlight professional skills and strengths by showing how these have been applied in previous positions or activities • Used when lacking a significant formal work history, yet with some activity that pinpoints talents, capabilities, and other professional assets
Combination	• When there is a mix or relative balance of professional skills/qualifications along with some work history • When neither the chronological nor functional style alone is more suitable
Entry-Level	• When little to no professional experience can be documented • To highlight education completed, technical skills mastered, practicum experience gained, certifications achieved, and previous volunteer work

and is identified by the position title for each entry. (Employers want to see *first* what you have been doing most recently in the workplace.) For each entry, the dates, or at least the month and year, are clearly shown, followed by the job title, company/employer name, job description, and accomplishments.

This type of resumé is best used by individuals who have a long, solid work history with minimal gaps between jobs. If a goal of the candidate is to demonstrate job stability, this is the optimal format. This type also accentuates position titles that are impressive or reflect great responsibility or leadership roles. Also, it highlights periods when the candidate may have worked with or for well-recognized or highly reputed employers. In certain situations, this type of resumé should not be used. Specifically, it is inappropriate when the candidate has a rather sporadic job history, when continuity of employment or involvement is lacking, or when the applicant has a long list of rather short-lived positions. In addition, this type of resumé is not useful for those in the process of making a career change, or in situations where the work history is irrelevant to the position sought. Figure 11-1 ■ contains an example of a (reverse) chronological resumé.

THE FUNCTIONAL RESUMÉ

The functional resumé can be thought of as a skills-based resumé. It accentuates the candidate's professional strengths, skills, and capabilities by showing where and how he or she has applied these in various positions or areas of specialty.

Those who lack any significant formal work history—perhaps young graduates seeking their first "real" job—should organize their capabilities and experiences in this format. Also, those who have been involved in various positions or functions in which professional skills and responsibilities

Thomas Moody, R.H.I.T., C.P.C.
1234 Sunnyside Dr.
Smalltown, FL 32851
Phone 352.421.1305 Email: tmoody43@anysite.com

Objective

To assist a hospital system in medical record compliance and in obtaining reimbursement optimally through proficiency in electronic claims procedures.

Employment History

March 2012–present   **Medical Records Technician and Billing Representative**
Sunnyside Family Practice, Smalltown, FL

- Evaluate and ensure accuracy of patient medical records
- Submit electronic claims utilizing Medical Manager
- Train new employees in administrative tasks

April 2008–March 2012   **Medical Billing Representative**
Medibill Solutions, Tampa, FL

- Utilized Medisoft program for claims submission
- Utilized ICD-9 and CPT-4 coding skills
- Assisted in office administration

May 2003–April 2008   **Medical Administrative Assistant and Transcriptionist**
Janson Chiropractic and Wellness Center, West Town, VA

- Assisted with reception, patient check-in forms, and filing
- Transcribed office medical reports at 60 WPM
- Maintained office supply inventory

Summary of Qualifications/Credentials

Registered Health Information Technician	January 2010–present
Certified Professional Coder	July 2009–present
HIPAA course certification	May 2009–present

Education

A.S. Degree	Health Information Technology	Myers College	May 2009
Diploma	Medical Office Assistant	FL Career Academy	May 2010

Figure 11-1 ■ **Example of a chronological resumé.**

were applied and those with no particular career path should organize their resumé in this way. Clear-cut and precise words and statements must be used to communicate these qualifications. The functional resumé should *not* be used when actual achievements gained or talents applied in past positions may be perceived as ambiguous.

Generally, the functional resumé emphasizes skills and qualifications to compensate for a relatively short or undeveloped work history. Figure 11-2 ■ contains an example of a functional resumé.

THE COMBINATION RESUMÉ

The combination resumé combines the objectives of both the chronological and functional resumé types into a hybrid form, usually by first specifying the candidate's qualifications, skills, and accomplishments and then showing the chronological work history. This type of resumé can showcase the candidate's best professional attributes and employment history. When both of these areas

---

Phoebe Turner, C.M.A.
1550 Callaway Dr. #202
Sandy Shores, SC 88921
Phone 881-412-9001 Email: pturner@anysite.com

Summary of Qualifications
- AAMA Certified Medical Assistant-proficient in phlebotomy, injections, EKG, vitals, X-ray/patient education, medical billing, and front office procedures
- Leadership and supervisory skills
- Excellent time management in multitasking within fast-paced environment
- Efficient computer operation skills in Microsoft Word, Excel, and Access
- Typing speed 55 WPM

Experience
Medical Assisting
- Completed 300 externship hours-Oceanside Family Medicine, Sandy Shores, SC
- 150 hours front office/150 hours back office

Leadership/Supervising/Time Management
- Managed restaurant staff of 35 with high rates of customer satisfaction
- Supervised front desk staff of large law firm
- Served as Vice-President in homeowners association; participated with board members in making community improvements

Computer Performance
- Performed secretarial work within law firm office utilizing Microsoft Office suite programs, proving versatile for many computer tasks
- Produced professional legal documents at 55 WPM, contributing to overall paperwork efficiency

Employment History

Staff Manager	Oceanside Seafood Grill	April 2002–May 2006
Legal Secretary	Martin, Bland, and Associates	August 2009–March 2013

Education

A. S. Degree in Medical Assisting	Hillside Community College	May 2016
Office Administration Diploma	Technical Institute of Boca	October 2008

References available upon request

Figure 11-2 ■ **Example of a functional resumé.**

for any particular candidate will be impressive to an employer, this resumé format is advisable.

This format is beneficial when work history is varied, when practicum or volunteer experience is to be included, and while changing career fields. It is helpful in demonstrating how a person has exercised the transferable skills he or she claims to possess.

Transferable skills are those skills that are useful, beneficial, and applicable to a wide range of other professional positions. Some examples of appropriate terms include but are not limited to *planning and implementing*, *managing*, *supervising*, *designing*, *coordinating*, *multitasking*, *assessing*, *training*, *using computer skills*, and *presenting*. In using these terms, it is important to clearly show what tasks these skills were used to accomplish. A combination resumé should *not* be used when even partially relevant work experience is lacking or when specific skills, qualifications, and achievements are not identifiable.

Examples of Transferable Skills

Human Relations–Focused Skills

- Listening
- Motivating
- Counseling
- Cooperating
- Establishing rapport
- Supporting

Planning, Organizing, and Management-Focused Skills

- Analyzing
- Solving
- Identifying
- Forecasting
- Initiating
- Decision making
- Delegating
- Promoting
- Coordinating
- Evaluating
- Implementing

Communication-Focused Skills

- Reporting
- Interviewing
- Negotiating
- Writing and speaking effectively
- Presenting
- Leading staff meetings

Professionalism/Work Ability–Focused Skills

- Managing time effectively
- Being punctual
- Demonstrating dependability
- Meeting set goals
- Meeting deadlines
- Organizing
- Cooperating
- Attending to details

Figure 11-3 ■ contains an example of a combination resumé.

John Smith, C.Ph.T.
1221 33rd Street North
Perry, FL 54321
508-513-9800 / jsmith79@anysite.com

Objective
To contribute to hospital pharmacy productivity while advancing in technical skills and pharmacy staff teamwork and leadership.

Relevant Skills
- Professional competency in pharmacy technology–C.Ph.T.
- Retail pharmacy technical and customer service skills for 2+ years
- Small business management (inventory, accounting and financial management) for 7+ years
- Computer skills (Windows and MacIntosh programs) utilized in all positions held using spreadsheet, database, and word processing applications

Experience
8/2015–present: Pharmacy Technician; XYZ Pharmacy, Perry, FL
    Maintained inventory, verified customer insurance, filled prescriptions, observed quality control procedures, helped ensure superior customer service.

6/2007–9/2014: Manager; ABC Shipping, Tallahassee, FL
    Managed finances, inventory, and operations of small shipping company; maintained increasing revenues and profits steadily each year; ensured customer retention through customer satisfaction.

7/2003–5/2007: Customer Service Representative, TalkCom Telephone Service Co., Atlanta, GA. Addressed customer inquiries and complaints; collaborated with division management to help resolve customer issues; presented telephone package options to interested customers.

Education
| 2005 | A.A. degree in Business Management | Southern Community College |
| 2015 | A.S. degree in Pharmacy Technology | Health Sciences Technical Institute |

Figure 11-3 ■ **Example of a combination resumé.**

THE ENTRY-LEVEL RESUMÉ

For students entering the allied health industry as a first profession—that is, without prior work experience in any other industry—the resumé can be formatted to emphasize the skills and knowledge possessed despite this lack of experience. In this type of resumé, it is especially important to document the practicum experience. Other key details to include in this type of resumé are technical skills related to your chosen allied health specialty, certifications you have obtained as a result of your training, and any part-time, full-time, or volunteer positions you have held. Even if you perceive this bit of experience as useless in your pursuit of professional work, you should still document the experience as it shows that you were actively participating in the workforce (rather than sitting at home watching TV!). Overall, this resumé format provides details of the recent training you have completed and shows that you are focused on building a successful career from this starting point.

When presenting this type of resumé to prospective employers, keep in mind that your interviews become even more important. In light of less experience, interviewers may be more critical of your responses and interview etiquette than those of a candidate possessing five or more successful years of professional experience. Figure 11-4 ■ contains an example of a suitable entry-level resumé.

Including Allied Health Information in the Resumé

Regardless of the type of resumé used, the allied health candidate should also include some very specific and relevant pieces of information. First, include the title of the credential earned in the area of specialization. Some examples are the Certified or Registered Medical Assistant (CMA or RMA), Registered Health Information Technician (RHIT), Certified Professional Coder (CPC), Certified Pharmacy Technician (CPhT), and so on. This will clearly demonstrate competency.

Recent graduates with only practicum experience in the field should include technical and clinical skills within the field in which employment is sought. Any other supportive certifications and coursework such as BLS, CPR, and First Aid certification; HIPAA certification; phlebotomy certification; and EKG/ECG certification should be listed. Inclusion of all competency areas is of special importance when applying for jobs in allied health.

Recommendations for Resumé Formatting and Writing

The overall look and clarity of the resumé you provide will influence how you are perceived professionally by anyone who screens resumés and interviewees. When numerous resumés are collected by the employer, it is likely that only the best applicants (according to what is seen on the resumé) will be contacted for an interview.

Thus, you should view your resumé as your one and only application for an interview. If the resumé is sloppy, disorganized, or unappealing for any reason, the resumé screener may quickly discard it without another glance.

Emma Anderson
2000 Evergreen Ln
Orlando, FL 55555
Cell: 777-555-3333 Email: eanderson26@anysite.com

Objective

To obtain a position as a Medical Assistant in an accredited facility where my skills and education can be utilized.

Education

Souther Technical College, Orlando FL	Jan 2018
Associate of Science, Medical Assisting	GPA 3.58

Certifications

Certified Medical Assistant
CPR Certified

Skills

- Bilingual (Spanish)
- Microsoft Office
- Medisoft
- Proficient at taking vital signs
- Assisting with ADLs
- Skilled in phlebotomy
- Medication administration/injections
- Collection and processing of laboratory specimens
- Phoning/faxing in prescription refills to pharmacy
- Faxing referral information
- Scheduling appointments
- Chart documentation
- Filing/pulling medical charts

Experience

Oct 2017–Jan 2018 Medical Assistant Student Trainee	Orlando Health 300 hrs; Front and Back Office	Orlando, FL
Aug 2016–Present Hostess/Waitress	Chili's	Orlando, FL
Apr 2015–Jun 2015 Baker/Cashier	Stop & Shop	Allentown, PA
Aug 2013–Aug 2014 Assistant Manager	Luna's Bakery	Allentown, PA

References available upon request

Figure 11-4 ■ **Example of an entry-level resumé.**

Your goal should be to create an attractive, easy-to-follow, and organized resumé with wording that makes a good first impression concerning your skills, experience, education, and so on. The following lists highlight some aspects of formatting and writing that you should adhere to as you develop the look and feel of your resumé.

Appropriate Formatting

- The resumé must be pleasing to the eye and attractive to the reader.
- The resumé must be clear and easy to follow; this can be done with appropriate spacing, indentations, headings, and punctuation. It should not contain lengthy, detailed paragraphs that make the page look too wordy. Brief, bulleted lists showing highlights under each heading are effective and create an organized look.
- The font used for the resumé should be simple, with font size kept in the average range of 10 to 14 points. The use of fancy or stylish graphics and shading is unnecessary for allied health resumés. *Never* submit a handwritten resumé to an employer.
- The resumé should be printed on very light-colored or white, good-quality paper for in-person distribution.
- The design of the resumé should grab the reader's attention and draw it to the most important aspects the resumé is intended to highlight.

Appropriate Writing

- Use relevant power words from your profession and action verbs to clearly identify your capabilities and experiences.
- Be sure that your grammar and spelling are impeccable. If an employer views a resumé with even a few or minor errors of this nature, he or she will likely disregard the represented candidate.
- Use an appropriate, professional-looking e-mail address within the contact information area of the resumé. E-mail addresses using silly or vulgar words, slang terms, or inappropriate implications will not amuse resumé readers or potential employers and may actually cause them to discard your resumé.
- If your experience is irrelevant to the work you seek, list the appropriate transferable skills (such as those listed previously in this chapter) that link your professional attributes to your new area of expertise.
- Through your written expression of previous experiences and relevant skills or qualifications, create a professional image that matches the prestige and salary you desire.
- Prioritize according to significance the information that falls under each heading or position title.
- Sell the benefits of your skills and qualifications by including how your skills are of benefit to the potential employer.

Finalizing the Resumé

Once you have completed your resumé, ask a few other individuals, including the career resource professionals at your school, to critique the wording and format. Then make the appropriate adjustments. Always save an electronic copy on the hard drive of your personal computer and on an external disk and/ or cloud drive. Keep a professional binder, organizer, or folder handy with several copies of your resumé on good-quality paper.

The Cover Letter

Your overall goal for submitting a cover letter with your resumé is to stir up an employer's interest in you as a possible candidate for an open position, while adding a slight personal touch. Any cover letter for an allied health position should reflect that you have some experience, at least a practicum, as well as some formal education and training in the field you are pursuing. More important, though, you must strive to sell yourself by communicating what you are able to do for the employer.

For example, you should briefly explain how your skills can contribute to the efficiency, productivity, and mission or goals of the facility, hospital, pharmacy, or office, as well as how your experience and accomplishments in past positions will benefit this employer. Do not include very lengthy points, though. The reader will want to move quickly through your brief and concise cover letter.

The tone of the cover letter should be conversational. Avoid using what you think might be big and impressive words, as letters with too many terminologies and pretentious words or phrases are often quite unattractive to the reader. Be yourself, but use proper wording, spelling, and punctuation, with the personal touch of thought and creativity. An effective and impressive way to add this personal touch is to briefly describe how you can apply your personal or professional experience to help the company meet or exceed its goals. Try to be specific in aligning your abilities with the company's goals, which can be customer service oriented, production oriented, growth oriented, or efficiency oriented, among others. Mentioning this in the cover letter will demonstrate that you have put thought into this company even before an interview and will highlight a portion of your personal qualifications for the position, which the potential employer will find quite impressive.

Always keep an electronic copy of your cover letter accessible so that you can alter the name and company/organization to which the letter is directed. You can also easily modify the letter as necessary when applying to several different employers. Figure 11-5 ■ provides an example of a cover letter.

Applying for Jobs

Once the resumé and cover letter are created, the application process can begin. Most of the time, job applicants will be required to submit their resumé

Ralph Taylor
222 East Main St.
Chicago, IL 60601
(312) 555-1212

May 20, 20XX

James Stark, M.D.
1450 N. Devonshire
Chicago, IL 60611

Dear Dr. Stark:

This letter is in response to your recent advertisement in the May 19, 20XX, *Chicago Sun News* for a certified medical assistant.

I believe that my qualifications are a good match for your position. During my medical assisting program at Central State College in Hometown, Illinois, I maintained a 3.6 GPA on a 4.0 scale.

My medical assisting program at Central State College was completed in December 20XX. I passed the American Association of Medical Assistants' certification examination January 27, 20XX. Currently I am completing an associate degree program at CSC and plan to graduate in June 20XX.

The enclosed resumé includes my experience as a part-time nursing assistant for Dr. Jane Young in her family practice office.

I look forward to meeting you to discuss your position needs and my qualifications.

Thank you for your consideration.

Sincerely,

Ralph Taylor

Ralph Taylor, C.M.A.

Figure 11-5 ■ **Example of a cover letter.**

and cover letter electronically, whether through e-mail, online job board, or the Web site of the company or organization. Exceptions to this are found in cases such as career fairs or direct referrals where an applicant is personally introduced to a hiring manager; in such cases, applicants would present in person with their documents. Many companies contract with job search Web sites to post their available positions, and many also maintain a career section within their company Web site. For job seekers, it is often most efficient to use popular job search Web sites (such as CareerBuilder.com, ZipRecruiter.com, Indeed.com, Monster.com, LinkedIn.com, and others) because many similar positions within the specified career field within a defined geographic area can be searched instantly. These Web sites typically offer job seekers free accounts; they enable users to search for the latest job postings, receive alerts about new postings, save their resumé and cover letter for easy applying, connect with employers via messaging in some cases, and use other helpful features.

When you find a job posting that appears to be a strong match for your career interests and your qualifications, follow the application instructions specified. Not all postings will include the same instructions. Some jobs can be applied for directly through the job search site where you first see the posting; others can be applied for by following a provided link to the hiring company's career Web page specifically for that position, where direct application and/or resumé submission can be made. Once you follow all steps of the application process and make your final submission, usually a confirmation statement appears to verify that you have successfully applied. Sometimes the company's career site will send an automatic confirmation email. It is advisable to apply for as many positions as possible for which you believe you are a good match. Finally, keep track of the positions and companies/organizations to which you have applied so that you remember and are prepared in the event that you are contacted to proceed with interviews.

The Waiting Period

The waiting period refers to the time between submitting your resumé in response to a job posting and receiving a response to your expressed interest. Keep in mind that waiting periods can vary, as different employers are operating on their own unique time frames for filling their position(s). You have a few issues to consider during this time.

Phone Contact

One very important fact is that an employer may contact you, most likely by phone, at any time. In the current age of high-tech smart phones, voice mails that play musical messages, music clips that play for callers while they await call pickup, and the like, many young adults and even older adults are fascinated by this technology and subscribe to these services. Although these are fun and amusing products of our time, they are *not in the least* fun *or* amusing to potential employers who are contacting you for a professional interview. What do you suppose an employer would think or do when greeted by a recording that plays a clip from a questionable rap song? Suppose the voice-mail message sounds something like "Yeah, hey, I ain't here now; leave a message," with audible TV and other background sounds muffling the entire message. How would this caller respond as a potential employer of a candidate who offered such a message? A highly likely response would be to hang up the phone and move on to the next candidate. Therefore, it is very important for your professional image during this job search phase to come across as mature and professional to anyone who contacts you. A simple message—such as "Hello, you have reached the voice mail of John Doe. Please leave a message. I will return your call as soon as possible. Thanks."—will be much more acceptable and respectable.

Another very important aspect of phone contact is the content and tone of the voice message you leave for the prospective employer, hiring manager, or interviewer. In speaking to this person's voice mailbox, it is necessary to maintain the same level of professionalism as you would in person. This means speaking clearly, politely, and with good intention. In other words, you do not want to come across as unclear or difficult to understand, lacking good manners, or sounding impatient or rude. Be prepared before calling by having an idea of how you will state your message in case the person is unable to take your call at that time. How you come across on the phone is another way the hiring manager or interviewer can in part determine your capability for a practicum or permanent employment, and thus, this should be a strong point.

E-Mail Contact

The next most popular form of communication from a potential employer is e-mail. The first and foremost point with using e-mail as an available line of professional contact with potential employers is to offer a decent, professional-sounding e-mail address with your contact information, as briefly mentioned already in the section on resumé writing. Creative, amusing, and sometimes even vulgar language references are common today in many people's personal e-mail addresses, but you must avoid these if you are hoping to be selected for an interview. If you currently use a not-so-professional e-mail address, sign up under a respectable name for one that can be used for professional correspondence throughout your life. For example, a first initial and last name or some variation of your name and a meaningful number would be appropriate.

Examples of Unprofessional E-Mail Addresses

- babygotback@somedomain.com
- chick4you@somedomain.com
- foreverhigh@somedomain.com

Such e-mail addresses are inappropriate because they all have vulgar intention built into them. Although this may be fun for strictly social contacts, such addresses must *not* be used for professional contacts.

Examples of Professional E-Mail Addresses

- kjcharles@somedomain.com
- becky43@somedomain.com
- jenna_bosworth@somedomain.com

Basic, straightforward, and unquestionable in nature, such e-mail addresses are acceptable and expected of employers seeking allied health professionals.

Also to be considered are the content, tone, and professionalism within any e-mail contact you make with the site manager or interviewer. This encompasses not only *what* you say, but also *how* you say it. Care must be taken to deviate from the format of common and informal e-mail and text messages we might typically send to family or friends and to compose professional messages using unabbreviated words, complete sentences, letter format (proper greeting and closing), and terms of respect. Tactics to avoid within professional e-mail messages are abbreviated wording, texting lingo, the absence of a greeting and closing with electronic signature, and any language that comes across as disrespectful or inappropriate. Always be sure to proofread the entire message before sending, making sure it reflects your intended meaning and purpose and that it is free from spelling and grammatical errors (check for correct capitalization, punctuation, sentence structure, etc.).

Familiarity with Organizations to Which You Have Applied

Spend time researching the companies or health care practices to which you have submitted your application and resumé. The best and most convenient resource is the company or office Web site. (Individual physician offices are less likely to have a fully detailed Web site available than are larger organizations, such as hospitals, large health care groups or chains, insurance or managed care organizations, and pharmacies.) In the rare circumstance that a Web site is unavailable, phone or stop by the location and ask for a business card, for a brochure, and for any other informative literature about the organization. Taking these actions during your waiting period will ensure that you are prepared for an interview, can speak intelligently concerning the respective organizations, and can ask meaningful or insightful questions when prompted during the interview. This indefinite time of waiting should not be wasted. Use it to your advantage.

Establishing and Fine-Tuning Your LinkedIn Profile

LinkedIn.com has become a widely used online resource in the professional world, encompassing all industries and professions. It is almost expected in current times that any individual serious about his or her career growth has an established LinkedIn presence. Fortunately, the basic service is free to users and provides invaluable benefits. During the waiting period is an excellent time to set up a new LinkedIn profile if you do not already have one. If you do have one, it is an excellent time to review and refine your profile to maximize exposure to the professional *you*.

First and foremost it is necessary to fully complete your profile. If you are hoping to gain recognition by other industry professionals or employers, a complete profile will be much more effective than a partially completed one. Once your profile is complete, you can start building your network. The best place to begin is simply with friends, family, and previous or current co-workers who also are active on LinkedIn. Because you have completed or are in the process of completing the practicum, it is of great benefit to connect with as many professionals from your practical training site as possible. This is especially important if your practicum is or was your first point of entry into the health care setting, so that you are connected to at least several professionals in your career field. From these starting points, LinkedIn will suggest new connections for you, and you have the potential to increase your network significantly over time.

Another way to greatly benefit from LinkedIn is by using the job search feature offered by the network. Like most other job search Web sites, LinkedIn allows users to specify position type and location criteria, then returns results for open positions. Many employers use this avenue to advertise job vacancies; it includes either a direct link to the employer's career Web site to apply for the specific position or to the Easy Apply feature (applicable to many posted positions) that directly pulls applicants' LinkedIn profile information and designated resumé file and submits them directly to the employer/hiring manager. As an aspiring allied health professional, using these basic features offered by LinkedIn will provide you a simple and effective way to enhance your professional networking efforts as well as to search and apply for jobs in your field.

The Interview

You will make your real first impression on a potential employer during the interview—and it's important that it be a good one. You should be mindful of your attire, as well as your etiquette, when preparing for the interview.

Dressing for the Interview

Professional attire and an overall professional appearance are necessary for a successful interview. As mentioned in Chapter 3, when attending a practicum interview, it may be appropriate to wear the scrubs that are normally considered your school uniform. This is not the case when interviewing for a professional job beyond the practicum. A business suit is appropriate for such an interview. For women, a business dress or business skirt and top with professional blazer are also appropriate.

Suits for interviews should be dark or neutral in color, well coordinated, and worn with appropriate dress shoes. Brightly colored suits or those with dramatic designs or prints should not be worn. Shoes should be neat, new in appearance, clean, and conservative in style.

Plan your interview attire so that you are sure everything is clean and pressed before the big day. Do not wear perfume on the day of the interview. Jewelry should be conservative, if worn at all: neat and moderate, not bold, big, or high-fashion. Remove jewelry or piercings beyond the ear lobe (e.g., upper ear, nose, eyebrow, and tongue). Hair should be clean and styled neatly; avoid a high-fashion or dramatic hair design for the interview. Keep in mind that outrageously colorful highlights or hair color such as pink, blue, or green will automatically tell the interviewer to not take you seriously. Candidates with visible tattoos and untraditional piercings may send this message as well. Be sure to carry a professional-looking binder or folder containing additional copies of your resumé and cover letter.

Etiquette for the Interview

It is important to make the best impression possible during your interview. The following list highlights the various areas of interview etiquette that must be heeded to achieve the level of an expected and appropriate performance:

- Make a mental note of the name of your interviewer(s) so that you can offer thanks by name at the conclusion of your interview.
- Your efforts in making the best impression begin at the moment you arrive on the employer's property and last until the moment you leave. If you drive to the property, do not enter or exit the parking area with loud music or bass vibrating. Everyone near a window will look to see who is responsible.
- Cell phones should be off and out of sight from the time of your arrival until you leave the premises, including while you are waiting to begin the interview.
- Arrive approximately 10 minutes early. This will allow the employer and staff to notice before the interview begins that you are punctual. It also will provide time in case you are asked to complete any relevant forms or an application before meeting with the interviewer(s).
- Greet the interviewer with a pleasant smile and a firm handshake.
- Do not let your mind wander during the interview, even if the interviewer decides to give you a ten-minute detailed speech about the organization. Pay attention so that you can think of good, quality questions to ask the interviewer when appropriate.
- Maintain eye contact. Do not stare into space or look around, especially at your watch or the clock, during the conversation.
- Sit upright with good posture. Do not slouch or lean on your elbows.
- Answer the question asked. Do not extrapolate, bringing other insight or answers to questions that were not asked. Some questions will require simple, straightforward responses, and some will require explanations and examples.
- Use good manners, saying "Please," "Thank you," "Excuse me," and so on.
- Avoid filler words that make you sound uncertain of what you are trying to say, such as "uh," "like," "you know." Keep your language simple. Do not try to use big words that are unnatural in conversation. Use technical terms only if the question asked requires you to use them to answer appropriately.
- Express confidence and competence throughout the interview, but do not brag or act haughtily.

At the end of the interview, thank the interviewer(s) by name and end with a firm handshake.

Nontraditional Approaches: Phone and Video Interviews

Thanks to technology as well as the need for greater efficiency in considering qualified applicants, some employers are now using new modes of interviewing—that is, phone interviews and video interviews. In the event that any of your potential employers chooses one of these methods as part of their interviewing process, it is important that you are as prepared as you would be for a face-to-face interview.

When it comes to the phone interview, you may feel tempted to think that this is a more casual event than a traditional interview. Although the benefits to you of this format include not having to dress professionally or use time and resources to physically go to the employer's site, park, and arrive on time, the professional factor should not be neglected. Because the interviewer will not be spending time with you in person, it becomes even more important for you to convey your professional qualities effectively through a phone conversation. The following should be considered for phone interviews:

- Be ready for your phone interview 5 to 10 minutes before the appointed call time.
- Be sure your surroundings are perfectly quiet. There should be no background noise, including voices, TV, music, or anything else that the interviewer may hear through the phone or that may cause distraction to you as you focus on the conversation.
- Be mindful of your tone of voice. Your verbal communication should come across as respectful and professional.
- Answer the interviewer's questions the same as you would in a face-to-face interview. Do not be tempted to provide quick, abbreviated answers simply because of the phone factor. Fully address the question asked; the interviewer will be listening for the same quality in your response as would be given in person.
- Thank the interviewer by name at the conclusion of the call.

The video interview format, on the other hand, entails more detailed consideration and preparation than the phone interview, and it can have varying levels of similarity to a face-to-face interview, depending on how it is conducted. Aside from physically going to the interviewer's office site, all other major interviewing rules and tips apply when it comes to the video interview. Video interviews can take place live (face-to-face, online), or they can be arranged to record your responses to prerecorded questions asked by the interviewer. In most cases you will use your PC's Web cam to engage in this method. The following should be considered for video interviews:

- It is imperative that you test your technology before the interview. Be sure you know how to use your Web cam, and ensure it is working within the hour before your scheduled interview time. Also ensure adequate lighting and clarity in the space where you will be situated for the interview.

- It is imperative that you appear the same as you would for an in-person interview. Therefore, dress in appropriate interview attire and present yourself as neatly groomed.
- If you have not had substantial practice using self-video technology in professional situations, it is advisable that you practice looking at your self-facing camera while speaking. That way you can become accustomed to seeing yourself as you respond to questions without becoming distracted.
- Arrive on time to your video interview. Be completely ready to begin approximately 10 minutes before the appointed interview time, and be situated at your computer with the Web cam prepared for recording. If your interview is a prerecorded question format to be completed "at your convenience" by a specified deadline, submit your interview session well in advance of the deadline, if possible.
- Listen intently to the questions asked and respond the same way you would in a face-to-face interview. The interviewer will tune in to how you respond and your overall professional demeanor, so show the best of your professional side. If the interview is live, make sure to look at the interviewer while speaking, make eye contact, and avoid looking at your reflection in the self-facing camera lens (if applicable).
- Be sure to thank the interviewer by name upon the completion of the interview.

The Thank-You Letter

The appropriate time to send a thank-you letter to the person(s) who conducted the interview is within twenty-four hours of an interview. This letter should first thank everyone to whom it is addressed for taking the time to meet with you, to discuss more about their organization and its needs, and to discuss your qualifications. Mention some aspect of the company or its needs that were discussed with you during the interview, and reiterate how that aligns with your interest, capabilities, and professional goals. If you would like the interviewers to know something relevant that was not mentioned in the interview, briefly mention it, as long as it ties into your statements and demonstrates a solid professional match between the organization and you. Before closing the letter, restate your appreciation for being considered for the position. With a thoughtful thank-you letter, you will add to the good impression you have already made. Figure 11-6 ■ provides an example of a thank-you letter.

In some instances of following up with a special thank-you to the interviewer, it may be appropriate at times to use e-mail, or possibly a text message, to accomplish this purpose in a way that is as effective as a traditional printed letter. As time passes and communication technology becomes more efficient, reliable, and acceptable in the professional world, many administrators, managers, doctors, department supervisors, and so on are relying

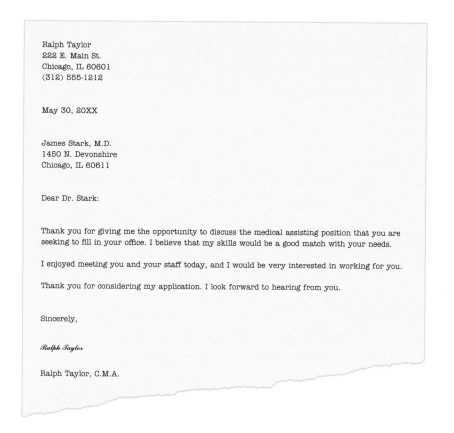

```
Ralph Taylor
222 E. Main St.
Chicago, IL 60601
(312) 555-1212


May 30, 20XX


James Stark, M.D.
1450 N. Devonshire
Chicago, IL 60611


Dear Dr. Stark:


Thank you for giving me the opportunity to discuss the medical assisting position that you are
seeking to fill in your office. I believe that my skills would be a good match with your needs.

I enjoyed meeting you and your staff today, and I would be very interested in working for you.

Thank you for considering my application. I look forward to hearing from you.


Sincerely,


Ralph Taylor


Ralph Taylor, C.M.A.
```

Figure 11-6 ■ **Example of a thank-you letter.**

on these methods for quick communication with their colleagues and others, especially when away from their office desks. In general, a professionally developed e-mail is acceptable for sending the thank-you letter, especially if the interviewer has provided you with his or her e-mail address. In composing this, be sure the message looks and reads as it would if it were provided in the traditional printed format. A text message thank-you is appropriate in cases where it is obvious that this type of communication is acceptable and embraced by the interviewer. For example, if the interviewer had previously made any contact with you via texting in discussing the position or scheduling the interview, then you automatically know that this method is accepted, maybe even preferred, by this individual. If the interviewer ever mentioned something to the effect of "If you think of any other questions, feel free to send me a text," then it is safe to assume that a text message thank-you will be appropriate. Take note however that when it is obvious that a text message is appropriate, the message still should be composed and worded professionally, with proper spelling and grammar; no texting lingo or abbreviations should be used, as this will diminish the professional quality of the message.

HIGHLIGHT

TIPS FROM PROFESSIONALS

On your interview day, you should strive to be your professional best to make a great first impression. You should arrive early, wearing appropriate professional attire and presenting with an extra copy of your resumé. During your interview, use good communication etiquette such as making eye contact and making sure you directly address the questions asked. When you answer questions, it is good to briefly explain your answers, but also to make sure you are not long-winded. Overall your conversation should reflect your interest in the job and in the interviewer. Finally, it is very important to thank the interviewer for taking the time to meet with you. It is advisable to send a follow-up thank you note (or email), as this again reinforces your appreciation and level of professionalism.

–Health Services Director, County Health Services

Spotlight on All Allied Health Specialties: Highlighting Practicum Experience on the Resumé

Many allied health students completing the practicum face the challenge of possessing minimal experience in the field to document on their resumé. It is common for hiring managers in health care to seek out candidates with some level of experience. For this reason, it is necessary for those without substantial health care experience to document their practical experience within the content of their resumé. Doing so will demonstrate completion of a structured training program and supervised practicum driven by specific performance objectives. The way to include the practical experience on the resumé depends on the format and style of the resumé. The content of the practicum experience should be included where relevant experience and/or training will be listed. The dates of the practicum, the number of hours completed, the name of the site, the location (city and state), and an overview of the main procedures and skills practiced should all be documented clearly.

Conclusion

As you have now observed, searching for employment is almost a full-time job. You can optimize your opportunities by first becoming familiar with your local job market and resources for scouting available positions in your allied health specialty. Carefully formulating your resumé to reflect the best possible professional image of yourself is of primary importance because in most cases your resumé is the first representation of you that employers will see. An impressive cover letter expresses your interests in the employers to whom you are submitting your application, while demonstrating your compatibility for the position and your abilities that will meet the employer's needs.

The interview is your time to shine. Prepare to make your best impression and to demonstrate confidence. Follow up the interview with a brief but meaningful thank-you letter to show your appreciation for the interview opportunity and to reiterate your interest in the available position.

Self-Prep Questions

In addition to considering the following questions as you prepare for your job search, review the Self-Prep Questions in Chapter 3:

1. List your most accessible resources for beginning your job search.

_____

_____

_____

_____

_____

2. Which type of resumé is most effective for you personally, considering your work history, education, practical training, volunteer activity, and so on? Why?

_____

_____

_____

_____

_____

3. New allied health graduates come from diverse employment and educational backgrounds. List at least three transferable skills from your work history or other activities that will be useful to mention on your resumé and during interview(s).

_____

_____

_____

_____

_____

4. List a few terms that you could choose from to briefly but concisely and effectively "sell yourself" in your cover letter. Be sure that these are supported by your actual accomplishments, and relate them to how they will likely assist the employer in achieving company goals.

_____

_____

_____

_____

_____

Role-Play Scenario

This scenario requires two individuals. One individual is an interviewer, and the other is a candidate for employment at an organization relevant to the candidate's allied health specialty. The group or class participating in this should plan the activity in advance so they can practice arriving to the interview on time, appropriately and professionally dressed, and with a resumé. Interviewers should gather appropriate interview questions from their school's career resource staff, from their instructors, or from researching interview questions on the Internet or other sources. Interviews should be approximately 10 minutes long (or more) for this activity.

1. In what ways has the candidate given a good first impression?

_____

_____

_____

_____

2. In what areas could the candidate improve to give a better impression?

_____

_____

_____

_____

_____

3. Based on the etiquette, appearance, and communication tactics employed by the candidate during the interview, what is your perception about his or her level of professionalism and ability to perform well in the prospective job?

_____

_____

_____

_____

_____

Readiness Checklist

_____ I understand that to be successful in the job search, I must be proactive in working through each step of the process.

_____ I know which local resources are most accessible and valuable to me in beginning my job search.

_____ I understand the importance of my resumé in capturing and holding the attention of potential employers.

_____ I understand the general differences among chronological, functional, combination, and entry-level resumés.

_____ I know which resumé format is most suitable for my use.

_____ I understand the meaning of "transferable skills."

_____ I realize the importance of appropriate formatting and writing for my resumé.

_____ I have thought of ways to "sell myself" in my cover letter by emphasizing how I can help my potential employer(s) accomplish organizational goals based on my own achievements and experiences.

_____ I understand the importance of using normal voice-mail messages during the waiting period, when I could be receiving responses from potential employers.

_____ I understand the importance of leaving voice-mail messages that sound appropriate and professional in my communication with prospective employers.

_____ I understand that written communication via e-mail with prospective employers should be professional and demonstrate respect.

_____ I understand the online job search and application processes.

_____ During the waiting period, I realize that I should spend time wisely by researching those employers to whom I have applied, so that I am well prepared for an interview at any time.

_____ I understand the appropriate style of dress required for an interview.

_____ I understand the various manners expected and those not to be exhibited during an interview.

_____ I understand the special circumstances of phone and video interviews, and how to perform well if presented with these interview formats.

_____ I understand that within twenty-four hours of any interview, I should prove my professionalism by sending the interviewer an appropriately written thank-you letter.

_____ I have saved or will save a copy of my resumé in electronic format so that I can easily update it when appropriate.

_____ I am prepared to succeed in the launch of my allied health career!

Appendix

Selected Allied Health Certification and Credentialing Resources

American Academy of Professional Coders (AAPC)

Credentials Awarded: CPC (Certified Professional Coder)
COC (Certified Outpatient Coder)
CIC (Certified Inpatient Coder)
CRC (Certified Risk Adjustment Coder)
CPB (Certified Professional Biller)
CPMA (Certified Professional Medical Auditor)
And more.
On the Internet: www.aapc.com

American Association of Medical Assistants (AAMA)

Credential Awarded: CMA (Certified Medical Assistant)
On the Internet: www.aama-ntl.org

American Dental Assistants Association (ADAA)

Professional organization in alliance with DANB
On the Internet: http://www.adaausa.org

American Health Information Management Association (AHIMA)

Credentials Awarded: RHIT (Registered Health Information Technician)
RHIA (Registered Health Information
Administrator),
And more.
On the Internet: www.ahima.org

American Medical Technologists (AMT)

Credentials Awarded: RMA (Registered Medical Assistant)
RPT (Registered Phlebotomy Technician)
RDA (Registered Dental Assistant)
CMAS (Certified Medical Administrative-Specialist)
MT (Medical Technologist)
And more.
On the Internet: www.americanmedtech.org

American Society of Anesthesia Technologists and Technicians (ASATT)

Credentials Awarded: Cer A.T.T. (Certified Anesthesia Technologist)
On the Internet: www.asatt.org

Association for Healthcare Documentation Integrity (ADHI)

Credentials Awarded: RHDS (Registered Healthcare Documentation
Specialist)
CHDS (Certified Healthcare Documentation
Specialist)
On the Internet: www.ahdionline.org

Association of Surgical Technologists (AST)

Professional Organization
On the Internet: www.ast.org

Dental Assisting National Board, Inc. (DANB)

Credentials Awarded: NELDA (National Entry Level Dental Assistant)
CDA (Certified Dental Assistant)
COA (Certified Orthodontic Assistant)
And more.
On the Internet: www.danb.org

National Board of Surgical Technology and Surgical Assisting (NBSTSA)

Credentials Awarded: CST (Certified Surgical Technologist)
CSFA (Certified Surgical First Assistant)
On the Internet: www.nbstsa.org

National Center for Competency Testing (NCCT)

Credentials Awarded: NCMA (National Certified Medical Assistant)
NCMOA (National Certified Medical Office Assistant)
NCET (National Certified ECG Technician)
NCPT (National Certified Phlebotomy Technician)
NCICS (National Certified Insurance and Coding Specialist)
And more.
On the Internet: www.ncctinc.com

National Healthcareer Association (NHA)

Credentials Awarded: CCMA (Certified Clinical Medical Assistant)
CPT (Certified Phlebotomy Technician)
CPhT (Certified Pharmacy Technician)
CMAA (Certified Medical Administrative Assistant)
CBCS (Certified Billing and Coding Specialist)
And more.
On the Internet: www.nhanow.com/home.aspx

National Registry of Emergency Medical Technicians (NREMT)

Credentials Awarded: Certified EMR (Emergency Medical Responder)
Certified EMT (Emergency Medical Technician)
Certified AEMT (Advanced Emergency Medical Technician)
Certified Paramedic
On the Internet: www.nremt.org

Pharmacy Technician Certification Board (PTCB)

Credential Awarded: CPhT (Certified Pharmacy Technician)
On the Internet: www.ptcb.org

Journal

Index